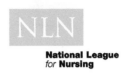

National League
for **Nursing**

Outcomes and Competencies for Graduates of Practical/Vocational, Diploma, Associate Degree, Baccalaureate, Master's, Practice Doctorate, and Research Doctorate Programs in Nursing

Developed by the National League for Nursing

National League for Nursing
61 Broadway
New York, NY 10006
212-363-5555 or 800-669-1656
www.nln.org

ISBN 978-1-934758-12-0

10 9

Art Director, Mara Jerman

Prnted in the United States of America

CD052022

Outcomes and Competencies for Graduates of Practical/Vocational, Diploma, Associate Degree, Baccalaureate, Master's, Practice Doctorate, and Research Doctorate Programs in Nursing

Developed by the National League for Nursing

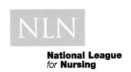

Table of Contents

List of Figures & Tables

Acknowledgments

The National League for Nursing thanks the following individuals for their contributions to the publication of this monograph: Meira Bengad, Leslie Block, Greg Clayton, Justine Fitzgerald, Bob Hartenstein, Mara Jerman, Karen Klestzick, Danielle Mackenzie, Angela McNelis and Barbara Spilka.

Preface

Recent years have witnessed significant, perhaps unprecedented, changes in health care in America. Change, of course, is a neutral word – a careful word, given the heated debates and passions that the topic of health care has lately given rise to. The problem is that these changes are neither unequivocally good nor bad. Few would turn back the clock and reverse the huge advances in medical research that have allowed so many individuals to live longer, healthier lives. Yet these very advances, along with larger societal factors (such as a declining birthrate, shifts in the workforce, and economic pressures), have created enormous challenges for the health care community today.

In response to these challenges, groups such as the Institute of Medicine (IOM), the Carnegie Foundation, and the National League for Nursing (NLN) have called for major revisions in the educational preparation of health professionals. Such calls charge the nursing profession to (a) articulate clearly what graduates of each type of program should be able to do, and (b) ensure that all graduates are well prepared to meet workforce needs and the needs of an increasingly diverse population.

Meeting this kind of challenge requires that nursing examine program outcomes and competencies across all types of programs – rather than looking at each program type in isolation from the others, as has been the case in previous work in this area. Such a comprehensive, inclusive approach serves to clarify concepts (e.g., evidence-based practice) that cut across all types of programs and, at the same time, clarify the unique focus of each program type in relation to each of those concepts.

Consistent with the NLN's commitment to excellence in nursing education, the NLN Education Competency Work Group was charged with specifying program outcomes and graduate competencies for each type of program – practical/vocational, associate degree/diploma, baccalaureate, master's, practice doctorate, and research doctorate. Education and practice members of this Work Group collaborated over a two-year period to review the literature, examine work completed previously by NLN advisory councils and work groups, formulate outcomes and competencies and vet them with the nursing education community, and finalize a set of outcomes and competencies that address all program types. The result was expected to be a comprehensive document that would be both contemporary and futuristic and that would fill a gap that had remained unaddressed despite previous attempts.

The publication presented here meets this goal. It addresses outcomes and competencies for each type of nursing program, and it reflects the NLN's core values of caring, integrity, diversity, and excellence. We hope that the material presented here will challenge nurse educators to design exciting curricula that position graduates for practice in a dynamic health care arena: practice that is informed by a body of knowledge and appropriate to each nurse's educational preparation; practice that ensures that all members of the public – individuals, families, groups, and communities – receive safe, quality care. Such curricula will bridge education and practice and advance the profession as a whole.

Foreword

As a landmark publication, this document lays the foundation for ensuring that all United States nursing programs can expand and develop while maintaining the highest standards of quality and excellence. Through a collaborative, collegial process, the authors have thoroughly reviewed both the classic and current nursing literature, and have examined present and emerging educational and practice trends. The result of their endeavors is an Education Competencies Model inclusive of all nursing program types. Nursing education is indebted to the committed volunteers and the various consultants who generously gave of their time and expertise to create this publication.

Do not be deceived by the brief length of this monograph. The authors have synthesized a huge amount of knowledge to create the first-ever comprehensive outcomes and competencies model for nursing education. All concepts came from the literature and were vetted by leaders in nursing education and practice, as well as through a national survey. The model incorporates long-held values (expressed, for instance, in the Code of Ethics of the American Nurses Association), as well as contemporary initiatives (such as quality and safety efforts promoted by the Institute of Medicine and other entities, including hospital-setting employers, over the last decade). The model appears simplistic but has hidden depth. It ensures that graduates will have assimilated the values, concepts, and ethical standards fundamental to nursing, and will have demonstrated competence in the skills and knowledge identified as central to nursing practice for each program. By adopting the model, nursing programs will assure their students, the public, nurse employers, and other nursing programs that graduates will have met a national standard.

This publication is a beginning. From here, nurse educators can differentiate between program types while assuming the responsibility to educate their students in what is valued and expected by the public and the profession. The model is not prescriptive; it is an invitation to explore and innovate, being always mindful of the consumer's and the profession's needs. The model is not a career ladder model, rather it supports the academic progression of all nurses entering the field. Likewise, it is not a licensure model. It is an academic model that embraces the multitude of educational institutions that prepare nurses. It is built around the American educational tradition and emerging trends, but it has global possibilities and application.

The health care reform effort in the United States is quickly emerging, through debates and legislation too numerous to mention. The year 2010 will be recognized as pivotal, similar to 1965, when the Medicare program for seniors was initiated. Yet it will take decades of quality initiatives to reengineer our practice environment. The model presented here launches nursing education into that preferred future, through guidelines that are broad, inclusive, and flexible. Present and future nurse educators can use the model to build curricula, further the science of nursing education, and explore and refine teaching, learning, and evaluation. In short, the model presented in these pages is a bold approach by nurse educators to stand shoulder to shoulder with employers and graduates to strengthen and revitalize our profession, while advocating for our nation's health.

Who we are and what we stand for must be addressed in every nursing program. As the voice of the profession to students, nurse educators bear this responsibility. The model presented here offers a framework to help nursing education meet this most vital goal.

The National League for Nursing proudly presents the first-ever comprehensive national model for nursing education. This historical document is the product of longstanding, persistent efforts, and the NLN's own core values of caring, integrity, diversity, and excellence. By embracing the model, nurse educators join the effort to develop the best-educated nursing workforce ever. America deserves as much.

Cathleen M. Shultz, PhD, RN, CNE, FAAN
President, National League for Nursing
Dean and Professor, Harding University College of Nursing

Section I: Introduction

Historical background

The National League for Nursing has long published competencies for graduates of nursing programs as guidelines to help faculty in different schools of nursing develop their curricula. Historically, these competencies were developed by the NLN's four education councils – the Council of Practical Nursing Programs, the Council of Diploma Nursing Programs, the Council of Associate Degree Nursing Programs, and the Council of Baccalaureate and Higher Degree Programs. Once a set of competencies was approved by a council, it was disseminated by the NLN to all members of that council and to the general public. While nursing schools used these documents to guide them as they developed, refined, and revised their academic programs, the competencies were never required as part of accreditation standards.

In the mid-to-late 1990s the education councils became somewhat dormant, and work on competency revision slowed. The Council of Associate Degree Nursing Programs did collaborate with the National Organization of Associate Degree Nursing (N-OADN) in 1998-1999 to prepare an updated version of competencies for graduates of such programs, and that document was published by the NLN in 2000 (under the title *Educational Competencies for Graduates of Associate Degree Nursing*). However, no other set of competencies was revised or updated after the mid-1990s.

As the NLN embarked on its path of revitalization in the early 2000s, the entire member involvement structure was revised, and the education councils were eliminated. This decision reflected the Board of Governors' goal to focus on larger educational issues that cut across program types. It also eliminated "silos" that tended to emphasize differences and program-specific issues that served only to isolate one program type from all others.

To replace these program-specific councils, in 2001 the NLN Board approved a new set of Advisory Council Executive Committees that were clearly aligned with the NLN's revised mission. NLN members were now invited to serve on the Nursing Education Advisory Council, the Nurse Educator Workforce Advisory Council, the Nursing Education Research Advisory Council, and other groups. Each of the new councils included elected members from various types of programs. Unlike their predecessors, which functioned largely as stand-alone bodies, the new councils were designed to work together within the overall NLN structure, and each was charged with addressing nursing education in its totality.

This new member involvement structure has served the NLN very well over the years, and it is still operational, though some new advisory councils have been added and the purpose and goals of others have been revised. In alignment with this success, the NLN recognized the need for an updated version of program outcomes and competencies for all types of programs. This proposal met with a groundswell of support from members of the NLN, schools accredited by the NLNAC (National League for Nursing Accrediting Commission), and organizations with which the NLN collaborates (e.g., the American Association of Community Colleges). With an eye toward the future, the NLN established the NLN Education Competency Work Group.

The Education Competencies Work Group

Since the work of developing program competencies was most closely aligned with the purpose and goals of the Nursing Education Advisory Council (NEAC), this group was charged with taking the lead in this area. The Work Group was comprised of all members of NEAC and various other individuals, including representatives from the practice arena and the QSEN (Quality and Safety Education in Nursing) initiative, as well as experts in nursing education. The inclusion of leading voices from both education and practice brought a dynamic perspective to the group, helping it reflect more comprehensively on emerging issues related to nursing, and on how best to prepare nurses who could meet the profession's future needs. This collaboration between education and practice reaffirmed for the Work Group that the purpose of nursing education is the *formation* (rather than simply the training) of nurses, and that this is a responsibility shared by both nursing education and nursing practice. (The full list of Work Group members is presented in Appendix A.)

In July 2008, the Work Group gathered for its first face-to-face meeting. The NLN's core values of diversity, integrity, caring, and excellence were prominent as the group began its work, as was the group's commitment to developing competencies that were inclusive of all program types and showed the relationships among them. Members agreed that to develop competencies for graduates of associate degree programs in isolation from those for baccalaureate programs, for example, would be nonproductive. Indeed, if a new list of competencies was to be useful, it clearly had to (a) show differences among program types, (b) show how competencies build from one program type to the next, (c) reflect contemporary nursing practice, and

(d) bridge the gap between education and practice. The Work Group's members further recognized that an emphasis on values, ethics, and the affective domain was critical for nurses practicing in today's and tomorrow's health care environments. The members agreed, therefore, that these foci must receive at least as much attention as cognitive and psychomotor dimensions as the competencies were being formulated.

Members of the Work Group conducted a comprehensive review of the literature related to both the concept of competencies in general, and to statements of competencies that had already been published. Through this literature review, the group ensured that it would not duplicate what other bodies had already done, and that it would produce an integrated set of competencies that would be comprehensive, inclusive, and measurable; show relationships among program types; and reflect the complexity of nursing education.

The Work Group carefully examined the following competency documents that had been published at the time of review:

- The American Association of Colleges of Nursing's *Essentials of Master's Education for Advanced Practice Nursing* (AACN, 1996)
- The AACN's *Essentials of Baccalaureate Education for Professional Nursing Practice* (AACN, 1998)
- Recommendations for the education of health professionals published by the Institute of Medicine under the title *Health Professions Education: A Bridge to Quality* (IOM, 2003)
- Dr. Christine Tanner's clinical judgment model (Tanner, 2006)
- The American Nurses Association's *Essential Nursing Competencies and Curricula Guidelines for Genetics and Genomics* (ANA, 2006)
- The core competencies drafted by the Massachusetts Organization of Nurse Executives under the title *Nurse of the Future: Nursing Core Competencies* (MONE, 2007)
- The program competencies developed by the Oregon Consortium for Nursing Education under the title *Competency Rubrics and Benchmarks* (OCNE, 2007)
- The quality and safety competencies of the Quality and Safety Education for Nurses (QSEN) initiative (Cronenwett et al., 2007)
- The TIGER (Technology Informatics Guiding Education Reform) recommendations regarding nurse informatics competencies (TIGER Informatics Competencies Team, 2008)

While each of these competency documents was carefully developed and all were valuable, none looked across all types of nursing programs in a comprehensive way, and many were too narrowly focused to meet the needs of the Work Group. The insights gained from reviewing these documents, however, did serve to inform members of the Work Group as they engaged in their task.

Formation of the Education Competencies Model

As a starting point for their work on the competencies, Work Group members were in agreement that a competency is a broad performance requirement related to the knowledge, skills, and attitudes needed by the nurse. (There is general support for this definition in the literature, though different terms may be used. "Knowledge," "skills," and "attitudes" are terms used by the QSEN initiative [Cronenwett et al., 2007]. Later parts of this monograph draw on the wording of Benner, Sutphen, Leonard, and Day [2009], who refer to skills as "practice know-how" and attitudes as "ethical comportment.") They were also in agreement that there must be a sound rationale for any competency that might be articulated. Finally, they agreed that outcomes (course and program) should be viewed as the endpoint of the successful integration of a set of selected core competencies for the particular course or type of nursing program.

During the initial period of review and preparation, which lasted many months, the Work Group explored a number of concepts that were evident in the literature. These areas included (but were not limited to) leadership, systems thinking, communication, collaboration, critical thinking, clinical decision making, evidence-based practice, innovation and creativity, global health, health care economics, ambiguity and uncertainty, and informatics. As they scrutinized and weighed different approaches, members of the group prepared numerous papers describing concepts and subconcepts, capturing salient information related to competency areas. Some of this work was deemed important, but ancillary, to the group's primary task. These items are presented in Appendix B.

After considerable review and discussion, it became evident that the concepts and subconcepts being examined clustered around six major areas, eventually referred to as "integrating concepts." These six integrating concepts are context and environment, knowledge and science, personal and professional development, quality and safety, relationship-centered care, and teamwork. Each will be discussed in turn later in this monograph.

Also during this period of review, the Work Group determined that a systems approach would be the most effective way of organizing and presenting its insights. Systems thinking is an approach to problem solving that sees each component of the system as integrated in the whole through a set of relationships and interactions. A systems perspective sees the system as being influenced by *inputs*, which are processed via *throughputs* to produce *outputs*.

Over time, a model emerged that placed the integrating concepts squarely within a systems perspective. The inputs were identified as the core values central to nursing education. These included the four core values of the NLN (caring, diversity, integrity, and excellence) plus three other values identified as fundamental by the Work Group – namely ethics, patient-centeredness, and holism. These seven values were identified as the foundation for competency development. The throughputs were identified as the integrating concepts named above – that is, the processes and concepts that are integral to nursing practice. The Work Group agreed that these concepts could be "horizontal," meaning always evident, or "vertical," meaning increasing in complexity as the nurse accumulates knowledge and experience.

Finally, the outputs were identified as the outcomes of the educational process – the skills, knowledge, and attitudes that graduates should have achieved upon successful completion of a program of nursing. The Work Group ultimately named four broad outcome areas as essential for graduates of all types of nursing programs: human flourishing; nursing judgment; professional identity; and a spirit of inquiry. The Work Group believed that while these outcome areas are few in number, they are comprehensive enough to encompass the whole of nursing.

Of course, the most important work was still to be done. For each integrating concept, the Work Group summarized the relevant literature, prepared a definition, and identified specific "apprenticeships" essential to that particular concept. Such apprenticeships are the areas of knowledge, practice, and ethical comportment necessary for learning a professional practice (Dr. Patricia Benner, personal communication, July 23, 2009; Benner et al., 2009). *Knowledge* encompasses the realms of science and theory. *Practice*, or "skilled know-how," refers to the ability to engage in the practice in a thoughtful, deliberate, and informed way; it is much more than the performance of technical skills. *Ethical comportment* means that an individual acts in accordance with a set of recognized values and responsibilities; it includes the notions of "good practice" and "boundaries of practice." This work culminated (through considerable generative thinking and reflection) with the formation of specific competency statements for each outcome, organized according to program type.

Once the outcomes and competency statements were in place, the Work Group developed a survey to solicit feedback from nurse educators and clinicians regarding their relevance, significance, and clarity. Feedback from the survey was then used to refine the material that is presented here.

The rest of this monograph is organized as follows. Section II offers an overview of the NLN Education Competencies Model and presents the model itself. Section III covers the core values (the inputs), Section IV the integrating concepts and apprenticeships (the throughputs), and Section V the outcomes and competencies (outputs). Section VI describes the survey and its results. The final three sections engage the reader in some of the broader implications of the model: ideas for education and practice partnerships (Section VII); implications of the model for the future of nursing (Section VIII); and recommendations for future work (Section IX).

Finally, a word about the language used in this document. New concepts and understandings in science require innovation and transformation in language. As in any dynamic and evolving discipline, a review of the literature in the science of nursing education reveals broadened definitions of traditional terms, along with new terms whose meaning is as yet unfixed. While terms such as *outcomes* and *competencies* may seem self-explanatory, small disparities in understanding relevant terms could lead to large disparities in understanding concepts. The definitions offered throughout this document (in the text proper and in a glossary, found in Appendix D) will ensure clarity and consistency of terminology as this model makes its way out into the world.

Section II: The NLN Education Competencies Model

Model development

When the NLN launched this project, it was in recognition that it is no longer sufficient to launch newly qualified nurses into the workforce armed only with mastery of a body of knowledge. We must instead prepare individuals grounded in values and ethics, with an understanding that knowledge is continually evolving, and with the skill to evaluate that knowledge and apply it in situations where nurses touch the lives of others.

It was clear throughout the development of the model that graduates of any type of nursing program should have several things in common. All nurses should be able to:

- provide safe care that is culturally and developmentally appropriate and that is centered on building and sustaining positive, healthful relationships with individuals, families, groups and communities;
- practice within a legal, ethical, and professional scope that is guided by accepted standards of practice;
- continually learn and grow as professionals whose practice is supported by evidence;
- advocate for access to and quality of health care.

It was also clear that the competencies across program types need to build in depth and scope, so as to promote educational progression and enhance the ongoing development of the nursing workforce. In other words, outcomes identified for graduates of practical or vocational programs should be foundational to outcomes for graduates of associate degree or diploma programs, and so on. While individuals who wish to pursue a nursing career do not need to begin in a practical or vocational nursing program, graduates of any program should have the knowledge and skill needed to progress academically. In this monograph, the competencies for each program type assume mastery of the competencies (or the foundational knowledge, skills, and values they express) previously assimilated.

The Introduction to this monograph describes how the Work Group elected to approach its task through a systems perspective, with the three main elements of inputs (here, the core values of nursing), throughputs (the integrating concepts), and outputs (program outcomes). Their work ultimately produced the NLN Education

Competencies Model, which is depicted in Figure 1. Each component of the model is described briefly here, and more fully explored in subsequent sections of this monograph.

Model components

The NLN Education Competencies Model graphically illustrates the dynamic process of mastering core competencies that are essential to the practice of contemporary and futuristic nursing. This multidimensional and multilayered model is revolutionary in design and adaptable to all types of nursing education programs. It affirms the unique characteristics of each type of program while promoting opportunities for multiple entry points. The model engages the nursing student and nurse educator in a transformative, proactive and collaborative encounter that represents an evolving and real-world experience in nursing education and practice.

The architecture of the model illustrates the personal, progressive, and lifelong professional development of the nurse through the accumulation, analysis, and synthesis of knowledge, scientific findings, and human experience. The model consists of the following components:

1. *Core Values:* Seven core values, implicit in nursing's historic paradigm, are foundational for all nursing practice. These values are *caring, diversity, ethics, excellence, holism, integrity,* and *patient-centeredness.* They are shown at the root of the model, to indicate that each type of nursing program and each type of competency must be grounded in each of these fundamental values.

2. *Integrating Concepts:* Emerging from the seven core values are six integrating concepts – namely, *context and environment; knowledge and science; personal and professional development; quality and safety; relationship-centered care; and teamwork.* These concepts are shown as bands around the program types, illustrating their progressive and multidimensional development in students during their learning experiences. The critical feature of the bands is an enveloping feedback mechanism that acknowledges the ongoing advancement of nursing education, as new graduates return new learning, gleaned from multiple sources, to nursing practice through nursing education. In this way, nursing practice and nursing education remain perpetually relevant and accountable to the public and all those in need of nursing.

3. *Program Outcomes:* The goals of nursing education for each type of nursing program can be summarized in four broad program outcomes. Nurses must use their skills and knowledge to enhance *human flourishing* for their patients, their communities, and themselves. They should show sound *nursing judgment,* and should continually develop their *professional identity.* Finally, nurses must approach all issues and problems in a *spirit of inquiry.* All essential program-specific core nursing practice competencies and course outcomes are subsumed within these four general aims.

4. *Nursing Practice:* Unbounded by any closed structures, the four program outcomes converge into nursing practice depending on the program type.

It should be noted that the model is an academic model, appropriate to all existing educational institutions that prepare graduates to work as nurses in the United States. The Work Group chose names and attributes that would permit them to use consistent, academic language to describe and differentiate between different program types. For example, programs that prepare vocational or practical nurses appear in high schools, vocational schools or institutes, single-purpose institutions, for-profit corporations, community colleges, and designated institutions of higher learning such as colleges and universities. The decision to call this program type "vocational or practical nursing education programs" precludes the need to differentiate between all the various organizations that prepare graduates for work as a practical or vocational nurse. Similarly, the Work Group chose to name the program types rather than use broad and confusing categories such as "prelicensure." The various types of programs are defined and described in Section V.

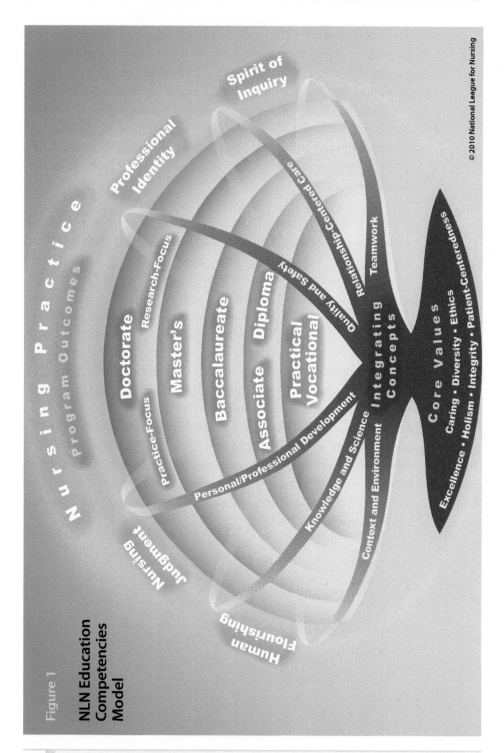

Figure 1

NLN Education Competencies Model

© 2010 National League for Nursing

Section III: Core Values

All types of work are grounded in a set of core values appropriate to that particular discipline, job, or pursuit. In nursing, our core values not only underlie our work, they are apparent in nearly everything we do, from the basic care provided by a vocational or practical nurse to the most advanced research and practice. All agree that a nurse should respect diversity in all forms; uphold given ethical and moral responsibilities; and strive for excellence while promoting holistic, patient-centered care.

The seven values described here include the four core values of the NLN (caring, diversity, integrity, and excellence) and three others (ethics, patient-centeredness, and holism) identified by the Work Group as fundamental to nursing.

Core values of the NLN

Caring. There is no question that caring is a significant and necessary dimension of nursing practice, regardless of the role assumed by the individual nurse. Nurses care for individuals, groups, and communities. They care for one another and themselves. And they work to create caring environments that promote the well-being of all. But what is caring? And what is a caring environment? While this concept has been defined in many ways by numerous experts, we used the following definition to guide development of the Education Competencies Model. (This definition, and the three that follow, are taken from the NLN [2007]).

> **Caring** means "promoting health, healing and hope in response to the human condition."
>
> "A culture of caring, as a fundamental part of the nursing profession, characterizes our concern and consideration for the whole person, our commitment to the common good, and our outreach to those who are vulnerable. All organizational activities are managed in a participative and person-centered way, demonstrating an ability to understand the needs of others and a commitment to act always in the best interests of all stakeholders" (NLN, 2007).

Diversity. Nursing takes place in a rich cultural climate, one that embodies the belief that nursing is for all, and that each person's worth and dignity is to be respected and valued. Valuing diversity means espousing inclusion and consideration of all persons as a framework for practice while meeting the needs of people around the world.

> **Diversity** means recognizing differences among "persons, ideas, values and ethnicities," while affirming the uniqueness of each.
>
> "A culture of diversity embraces acceptance and respect. We understand that each individual is unique and recognize individual differences, which can be along the dimensions of race, ethnicity, gender, sexual orientation, socioeconomic status, age, physical abilities, religious beliefs, political beliefs, or other ideologies. A culture of diversity is about understanding ourselves and each other and moving beyond simple tolerance to embracing and celebrating the richness of each individual. While diversity can be about individual differences, it also encompasses institutional and system-wide behavior patterns" (NLN, 2007).

Excellence. To define what excellence means for nursing may be impossible. Definitions, by their nature, are limiting; and excellence is seen not as a goal that can be achieved, but as an aspiration toward which we must continually strive. The pursuit of excellence means that no matter what standards are met, the status quo is never good enough. Improvement is always possible, and we must continually seek creative, bold, and original ways to do things better.

> **Excellence** means "creating and implementing transformative strategies with daring ingenuity."
>
> "A culture of excellence reflects a commitment to continuous growth, improvement, and understanding. It is a culture where transformation is embraced, and the status quo and mediocrity are not tolerated" (NLN, 2007).

Integrity. Integrity can be defined as striving consistently to do the right thing at the right time for the right reasons. In nursing practice, this means recognizing, with humility, the human dignity of each individual patient, fellow nurse, and others whom we encounter in the course of our work. It means recognizing that certain actions would compromise our own dignity as human beings and nursing professionals. It means accepting accountability for our actions while being fully committed to the betterment of patient care, and while advocating for patients in a consistently professional and ethical manner.

> **Integrity** means "respecting the dignity and moral wholeness of every person without conditions or limitation."
>
> "A culture of integrity is evident when organizational principles of open communication, ethical decision making, and humility are encouraged, expected, and demonstrated consistently. Not only is doing the right thing simply how we do business, but our actions reveal our commitment to truth telling and to how we always see ourselves from the perspective of others in a larger community" (NLN, 2007).

Additional core values

Ethics. Ethics encompasses the moral values and professional conduct inherent to nursing. Practicing ethically means distinguishing between right and wrong, and acting in accordance with the former.

The Work Group wrote the following definition of ethics to guide the development of the NLN Education Competencies Model.

> **Ethics** involves reflective consideration of personal, societal, and professional values, principles, and codes that shape nursing practice. Ethical decision making requires applying an inclusive, holistic, systematic process for identifying and synthesizing moral issues in health care and nursing practice, and for acting as moral agents in caring for patients, families, communities, societies, populations, and organizations. Ethics in nursing integrates knowledge with human caring and compassion, while respecting the dignity, self-determination, and worth of all persons.

Holism. Perhaps one of the things nurses do best is consider the patient as a complete human being. Holism embraces the belief that people are complex, dynamic, and not reducible to the sum of their parts. Nurses consider every aspect of the human condition when planning, implementing, and managing care for patients.

> **Holism** is the culture of human caring in nursing and health care that affirms the human person as the synergy of unique and complex attributes, values, and behaviors, influenced by that individual's environment, social norms, cultural values, physical characteristics, experiences, religious beliefs and practices, and moral and ethical constructs, within the context of a wellness-illness continuum.

Patient-Centeredness. Individuals become nurses so they may care for patients – that is, other human beings who happen to be ill or in need of care. Meeting the needs of patients means not just ensuring that they are kept comfortable and their dressings changed. It means recognizing that they (and their families) are autonomous beings, with needs and desires that deserve respect.

The following definition of patient-centeredness is drawn from Cronenwett et al. (2007).

> **Patient-Centeredness** is an orientation to care that incorporates and reflects the uniqueness of an individual patient's background, personal preferences, culture, values, traditions, and family. A patient-centered approach supports optimal health outcomes by involving patients and those close to them in decisions about their clinical care. Patient-centeredness supports the respectful, efficient, safe, and well-coordinated transition of the patient through all levels of care.

Section IV: Integrating Concepts and Apprenticeships

Nursing students must develop the ability to move with grace through the many realms of nursing. They must master varied areas of knowledge and science. They must be prepared to operate in complex environments while meeting the highest standards of quality and safety. They must be able to work comfortably in teams. And, with an awareness of their own personal and professional growing edge and learning needs, they must be able to build the relationships by which they touch and respond to those in need.

The Work Group deliberately chose the term *integrating concepts* for the ideas presented in this section. These concepts are not meant to be understood in isolation, rather as integrated within a whole. This notion is in keeping with our belief in holistic practice. The various strands all touch one another, even if the whole is grasped only imperfectly or incompletely throughout one's professional life.

In this section, each of the six integrating concepts (context and environment; knowledge and science; personal and professional development; quality and safety; relationship-centered care; and teamwork) is described, defined, and then further explicated by the knowledge, practice, and ethical comportment apprenticeships inherent to that concept. These apprenticeships offer a set of specific knowledge, understanding, and skills that nurses should become familiar with as they progress in their learning. The apprenticeships are deliberately general, rather than being divided according to the different program types. This is because, as noted in the Foreword to this document, the model presented here is not meant to be prescriptive. The model gives different programs room to explore and innovate, while supporting the academic progression of nurses from one program to another. The apprenticeships allow student nurses to develop an ever-widening lens of understanding and an expanding repertoire of dynamic response patterns. The integrative thinking that lies behind the model encourages the nurse to view unfolding, complex situations from multiple perspectives, apply different interpretative schemas while grasping the situation's salient elements, and respond in healing and healthful ways.

The three types of apprenticeships – knowledge, practice, and ethical comportment – are based on work by Benner et al. (2009), published under the auspices of the Carnegie Foundation for the Advancement of Teaching. As described in the Introduction, *knowledge* encompasses the realms of science and theory. *Practice* includes the mastery of technical skills and the notions of situated thinking and knowledge use; it means being able to engage in practice in a thoughtful, deliberate, and informed way. *Ethical comportment* involves the individual's formation within a set of recognized responsibilities; it includes the notions of "good practice" and "boundaries of practice."

A. Context and Environment

Context, in its simple definition, is the setting in which something happens; the circumstances that lie behind a situation or event. In relation to organizations, one can conceptualize context in terms of the conditions or social system within which the organization's members act to achieve specific goals (Blau & Scott, 1962; Etzioni, 1964).

Structural contingency theory (SCT) offers insights into organizational effectiveness and its relationship to context. The theory posits that context, for an organization, is comprised of three elements: the kind of work performed in the organization; its external environment (a product of factors like regulatory requirements and market conditions); and its internal environment (produced by the behaviors and interactions of organization members). The structure of an organization, according to this theory, is a product of the context within which the organization operates. Structure refers to the administrative components that are used to balance coordination and control of work with occupational and role specialization, so that the organization may better accomplish its goals. The basic principle of SCT is that there is no single best way to structure work in an organization to achieve effective performance and, hence, optimal outcomes. Rather, effectiveness depends on structuring the work in ways that are compatible with the organization's context (Donaldson, 1999).

The Work Group considered and integrated multiple subconcepts in formulating its understanding of context and environment (some of this work appears in Appendix B). The definition offered here builds on those subconcepts as well as on the insights of the scholars named above: Blau and Scott (1962) and Etzioni (1964) on context, and Donaldson (1999) and others who developed the SCT framework. It also draws from the ideas of Rathert and Fleming (2008) about the moderating role of strong leadership in creating both effective teamwork and an ethical climate in health care.

> Context and Environment, in relation to organizations, refers to the conditions or social system within which the organization's members act to achieve specific goals. Context and environment are a

product of the organization's human resources, and also the policies, procedures, rewards, leadership, supervision, and other attributes that influence interpersonal interactions. In health care, context and environment encompass organizational structure, leadership styles, patient characteristics, safety climate, ethical climate, teamwork, continuous quality improvement, and effectiveness.

Apprenticeships for Context and Environment

<u>Knowledge</u>
Nursing education should ensure graduates are familiar with concepts and literature in the following areas:

- Change, uncertainty, complexity theories; impact of continual knowledge explosion and constant evolution of technology; decision making in uncertainty; management of conflicting information; blurring of role boundaries and the resultant uncertainty about role expectations
- Codes of ethics (e.g., American Nurses Association, 2005; International Council of Nurses, 2006); regulatory and professional standards (ANA Social Policy Statement [ANA, 2003]; HIPAA [Health Insurance Portability and Accountability Act]); ethical decision making models; scope of practice considerations; principles of informed consent, confidentiality, patient self-determination
- Environmental health; health promotion/disease prevention (e.g., transmission of disease, disease patterns, epidemiological principles); chronic disease management; health care systems; transcultural approaches to health; family dynamics
- Health care economic policy; reimbursement structures; accreditation standards; staffing models and productivity; supply chain models
- American Association of Critical Care Nurses' six principles of a healthy work environment (AACN, 2005); regulations and legislation relevant to nurses' rights
- Functionality of clinical and financial systems (data entry, documentation, data retrieval); interoperability of systems; access and search of databases; shared languages; business rules and workflow management
- Components of creativity and creative processes; non-linear problem solving; innovation theory

- Leadership models (e.g., shared leadership, authentic leadership, transformational leadership)
- Systems theory; systems archetypes; system supports and barriers; methods of quality improvement; organizational theory; root cause analysis

Practice
Nursing education should ensure graduates are able to:

- Apply evidence to support decision making in situations characterized by ambiguity and uncertainty
- Apply professional standards; show accountability for nursing judgment and actions; develop advocacy skills; apply ethical decision making models
- Read and interpret data; apply health promotion/disease prevention strategies; apply health policy; conduct population-based transcultural health assessments and interventions
- Apply financial theories in practice
- Apply principles of a healthy work environment
- Navigate clinical and financial systems; manage health record information
- Employ brainstorming techniques; internalize a questioning pattern of thought
- Apply leadership models in practice

Ethical comportment
Nursing education should prepare graduates to:

- Analyze ethical challenges presented by ambiguous and uncertain clinical situations; self-assess one's own tolerance for ambiguity and uncertainty; accept the possibility of multiple "right" answers (rather than one-right-answer thinking) in patient care and other professional situations
- Examine personal beliefs, values, and biases with regard to respect for persons, human dignity, equality, and justice; explore ideas of nurse caring and compassion
- Show respect for others' values; appreciate diversity; be civil during relationships and work; value community empowerment and social justice; work to improve social conditions affecting health; adopt inclusive language
- Act in accordance with policies and procedures that guide economic behavior in the practice environment
- Act in accordance with legal and regulatory requirements, including HIPAA,

for faculty, students, patients, and families
- Value the importance of good leadership to optimal team functioning
- Appreciate the influence of systems on health care outcomes

B. Knowledge and Science

Nursing is a practice discipline that draws on knowledge from a large number of fields. Nurses must integrate knowledge from (a) the biological sciences (biology, chemistry, anatomy and physiology, microbiology, genetics, etc.); (b) the social sciences (psychology, sociology, epidemiology, family dynamics, community dynamics, etc.); and (c) the arts and humanities (writing, public speaking, history, religious studies, multicultural studies, women's studies, etc.). Thus, individuals preparing to be nurses learn theories related to human needs, learning, developmental stages, communicable disease transmission, and many other areas of human and community functioning.

In addition to drawing on knowledge from disciplines outside our field, nursing is developing its own science. Scholars of nursing, like their counterparts in more established disciplines, engage in an ongoing process of asking questions, conducting research, developing and testing theories, and integrating their research findings and theories into a systematic body of knowledge. Nursing science explores concepts that are relevant to our practice (from physiological functions to living conditions; from emotional strength to the transmission of pathogens) and explains the interrelationships among them (for instance, the inverse association between wellness and poverty). Through rigorous scientific investigations, nursing scholars test the hypotheses integral to the science and document best practices.

In developing the definition presented here, members of the Work Group were guided by the following understandings:

- **Disciplines outside nursing** refers to all those fields that relate to and support the practice of nursing, from medicine and pharmacology to social work, from physical therapy and nutrition to art and music. Men and women preparing to be nurses must learn and integrate into their practice a large body of knowledge from these disciplines. In addition, it is important for nurses to understand the roles of professionals in other health disciplines so that interdisciplinary collaboration can be most effective and collegial.

- **Nursing science** is the systematic body of knowledge about the practice of nursing. Nurse scientists ask questions about how best to identify and manage patient health problems, conduct research to enhance our understanding of nursing practice situations, develop and test theories about the relationships among concepts in our field, and integrate research findings and theories into a systematic body of knowledge. Repeated testing of hypotheses yields evidence that supports the practice of nursing and fosters nurse engagement in evidence-based practice (see below). Such practice helps create and sustain a culture of inquiry and quality.

• *Development of a science* refers to the ways in which the concepts central to a discipline are defined, interrelated, tested, compiled into a database, and so on. Each member of a discipline has some degree of responsibility for contributing to the development of its science, whether by designing rigorous qualitative and quantitative studies, or simply by approaching practice in a spirit of inquiry. Appendix C presents the NLN's Science of Nursing Education Model (2003), adapted for this document. The model illustrates the many activities that must be undertaken to develop a science and the many ways in which members of a discipline can contribute to the ongoing evolution of that body of knowledge.

• *Evidence-based practice*, according to Ingersoll's (2000) widely accepted definition, involves the conscientious, explicit, and judicious use of theory-derived, research-based information in making decisions about care delivery to individuals or groups of patients, in consideration of individual needs and preferences.

Knowledge and Science refer to the foundations that serve as a basis for nursing practice, which, in turn, deepen, extend, and help generate new knowledge and new theories that continue to build the science and further the practice. These foundations include (a) understanding and integrating knowledge from a variety of disciplines outside nursing that provide insight into the physical, psychological, social, spiritual, and cultural functioning of human beings; (b) understanding and integrating knowledge from nursing science to design and implement plans of patient-centered care for individuals, families, and communities; (c) understanding how knowledge and science develop; (d) understanding how all members of a discipline have responsibility for contributing to the development of that discipline's evolving science; and (e) understanding the nature of evidence-based practice.

Apprenticeships for Knowledge and Science

Knowledge
Nursing education should ensure graduates are familiar with concepts and literature in the following areas:

- What is (a) a science? (b) evidence-based practice (EBP)? (c) informatics?
- How (a) sciences, (b) the evidence on which practice is based, and (c) informatics are developed, and by whom; the relationships between research and science building, and between research and EBP
- The state of the science in nursing
- Relationships between knowledge/science and (a) quality and safe patient care, (b) excellence in nursing, and (c) advancement of the profession
- Integration of knowledge from nursing and other disciplines
- Elements of the research process and methods of scientific inquiry
- Electronic databases; literature retrieval; evaluating data for validity and reliability; evidence and best practices for nursing

Practice
Nursing education should ensure graduates are able to:

- Retrieve research findings and other sources of information; critique research to judge its value and usefulness; evaluate the strength of evidence for application of research findings to clinical practice
- Translate research into practice in order to promote quality and improve practices
- Systematically reflect on practice as a basis for the generation of new knowledge and innovation
- Design quality research studies as appropriate
- Use databases for practice, administrative, education, and/or research purposes; document via electronic health records; use software applications related to nursing practice

<u>Ethical comportment</u>
Nursing education should prepare graduates to:

- Value evidence-based approaches to yield best practices for nursing
- Appreciate that each and every nurse bears some responsibility to advance nursing knowledge and the science of nursing
- Maintain a questioning mind and spirit of inquiry; be open to new ideas and approaches
- Be willing to take risks and to make mistakes; be prepared to learn from mistakes
- Appreciate the importance of disseminating research findings

C. Personal and Professional Development

Nursing education is designed to prepare graduates who can function effectively as practical nurses, registered nurses, advanced practice clinicians, educators, administrators, case managers, researchers, and policy developers. To assume any one of these roles requires a sound base of knowledge and understanding in nursing and a variety of other disciplines that complement practice. Ensuring that graduates have a sound knowledge base for their practice – in whatever role – is not enough. Graduates also must demonstrate many personal and professional abilities and attributes that are essential for them to be most effective in their roles and as members of the profession. The process of refining and integrating these abilities and attributes is referred to as personal and professional development.

In attending to the personal and professional development of students, nurse educators and practicing nurses facilitate their growth and socialization (Halstead, 2007; NLN, 2005). Such education helps students understand and appreciate the complexity of the legal parameters, regulatory requirements, and ethical principles that guide nursing practice. It also helps students understand what it means to be a professional, the contributions nurses make to the health of our nation, how the role of the nurse has evolved over time and continues to change, and how nurses can help shape a preferred future for health care and the profession.

Personal and professional development includes training in effective communication skills. Communication may be therapeutic in nature and occur with patients and their families. It may be professional in nature and occur through one's contributions to interdisciplinary teams, committee participation, writing, or formal presentations. Finally, communication may be a key component of conflict resolution strategies.

Development as a professional also includes learning about leadership and how each nurse can take on the mantle of leadership, regardless of role or scope of responsibility. Leadership, in turn, incorporates innovation and creativity, being comfortable with ambiguity and uncertainty, caring for oneself, and pursuing lifelong learning, all of which must be addressed in the preparation of nurses.

> **Personal and Professional Development** is a lifelong process of learning, refining, and integrating values and behaviors that (a) are consistent with the profession's history, goals, and codes of ethics; (b) serve to distinguish the practice of nurses from that of other health care providers; and (c) give nurses the courage needed to continually improve the care of patients, families, and communities and to ensure the profession's ongoing viability.

Apprenticeships for Personal and Professional Development

Knowledge

Nursing education should ensure graduates are familiar with concepts and literature in the following areas:

- Creativity and creative processes
- Innovation and diffusion of innovation theories
- Codes of ethics and regulatory and professional standards (as described in the Apprenticeships for Context and Environment); ethical decision making models
- Change, uncertainty, and complexity theories
- Impact of continual knowledge explosion and constant evolution of technology
- Blurring of role boundaries and the resultant uncertainty about role expectations
- Leadership styles and strategies; difference between leadership and management

Practice

Nursing education should ensure graduates are able to:

- Identify problems
- Engage in non-linear problem solving (e.g., brainstorming, examination of multiple alternative possibilities); manage conflicting information
- Apply decision making skills, particularly in the context of uncertainty and ambiguity
- Apply advocacy skills and ethical decision making models
- Employ tools for conflict management; apply leadership skills

Ethical comportment

Nursing education should prepare graduates to:

- Be willing to take the risks inherent in creativity and innovation
- Be aware of personal beliefs, values, and biases
- Demonstrate respect for all persons, and for human dignity, equality, and justice
- Demonstrate caring and compassion
- Be willing to assume a leadership role when needed
- Accept multiple "right" answers (rather than engaging in "one-right-answer" thinking) in patient care and other professional situations; be accepting of uncertainty and ambiguity

D. Quality and Safety

In the past, quality and safety meant ensuring that the individual practitioner could be relied on to provide sympathetic and effective care based on sound principles of nursing. This paradigm worked in a world where nurses saw fewer patients, and patients fewer nurses. Today's health care environment – with its challenging patient populations, pressure on resources, regulatory demands, and an unstable job market for practitioners – demands an emphasis on system effectiveness to provide quality health care and a safe environment for patients and workers.

Recognizing the need for a new emphasis on a culture of safety, health care organizations and educational institutions have taken up the challenge. In 2001, the Institute of Medicine established a new set of competencies for health care professionals: patient-centered care; teamwork and collaboration; evidence-based practice; informatics; and quality improvement. The IOM identified the components of quality care as safe, effective, patient-centered, timely, efficient and equitable, with safety the foundation upon which all other aspects of quality care are built. Later, the Quality and Safety Education for Nurses initiative brought together leaders in nursing education, nursing practice, and medicine to adapt the IOM competencies for nursing. The QSEN added safety to the list of IOM competencies, bringing the total to six.

The definition and apprenticeships below build upon the work of the IOM and QSEN. The IOM defines quality as the degree to which health services to individuals and populations increase the likelihood of desired health outcomes and are consistent with current professional knowledge (IOM, 2001). The QSEN *safety* competency requires that nurses minimize risk of harm to patients and providers through both system effectiveness and individual performance (Cronenwett et al., 2007).

Key to the apprenticeships is the insight that the most critical role of today's nurse is to provide essential leadership and accountability for patient safety across all health care settings – that is, coordinating and ensuring quality within the care directly provided by nurses and across care delivered by others (Mitchell, 2008). New graduates need to understand and value the importance of a systemwide safety culture, to advocate for open reporting, to learn from diverse events, and to report hazards and adverse events (Sherwood & Drenkard, 2007).

> **Quality and Safety** is the degree to which health care services 1) are provided in a way consistent with current professional knowledge; 2) minimize the risk of harm to individuals, populations, and providers; 3) increase the likelihood of desired health outcomes; and 4) are operationalized from an individual, unit, and systems perspective.

Apprenticeships for Quality and Safety

Knowledge

Nursing education should ensure graduates are familiar with concepts and literature in the following areas:

- Informatics
- Policies and procedures
- Current best practices

- Tools for effective and open communication
- The shortcomings of the human memory
- Sentinel events and root cause analysis; system effectiveness
- Factors that contribute to a systemwide safety culture; the importance of reporting hazards and adverse events; the "just culture" approach to system improvement

Practice

Nursing education should ensure graduates are able to:

- Communicate potential risk factors and actual errors
- Communicate effectively with different individuals (team members, other care providers, patients, families, etc.) so as to minimize risks associated with handoffs among providers and across transitions in care
- Encourage patients and families to communicate their observations and concerns regarding safety
- Use technologies that contribute to safety
- Carefully maintain and use electronic and/or written health records
- Stay current in professional health care knowledge
- Contribute to assessment of outcome achievement

Ethical comportment

Nursing education should prepare graduates to:

- Engage in lifelong learning to keep professional knowledge current
- Promote communication and open reporting as a priority in health care
- Commit to a generative safety culture
- Appreciate the cognitive and physical limits of human performance
- Value and encourage nurses' involvement in the design, selection, implementation, and evaluation of information technologies to support patient care (e.g., as recommended by QSEN)

E. Relationship-Centered Care

The relationships of health care practitioners with their patients, their patients' families and communities, and other health care providers are central to providing health care that integrates caring, healing, and community. Relationships with individual patients demand attention to each person in all of his or her complexity

– especially to the meaning of health and illness to the individual. Indeed, the very notion of a relationship presumes that the "other" is viewed as a person, not simply an illness. Relationships practitioners form with the communities they serve, as well as with other practitioners with whom they work, are equally important. Thus, a focus on ways to enhance and enrich relationships that are relevant to health care can only enhance the practice of nursing (Trosolini & Pew-Fetzer Task Force, 1994).

> **Relationship-Centered Care** positions (a) caring; (b) therapeutic relationships with patients, families, and communities; and (c) professional relationships with members of the health care team at the core of nursing practice. It integrates and reflects respect for the dignity and uniqueness of others, valuing diversity, integrity, humility, mutual trust, self-determination, empathy, civility, the capacity for grace, and empowerment.

Apprenticeships for Relationship-Centered Care

Knowledge
Nursing education should ensure graduates are familiar with concepts and literature in the following areas:

- The self as a resource
- The role of family, culture, and community in a person's development
- Factors that contribute to or threaten health
- Effective communication
- Threats to the integrity of relationships, and the potential for conflict and abuse
- Health care approaches of other disciplines and other cultures; power inequities across health care professions
- Team building and team dynamics

Practice
Nursing education should ensure graduates are able to:

- Engage in self-reflection
- Learn continuously, derive meaning from others' work, and learn from experience within the health care community; learn cooperatively; facilitate the learning of others

- Communicate information effectively; listen openly and cooperatively
- Promote and accept the patient's emotions; accept and respond to distress in patient and self; facilitate hope, trust, and faith
- Share responsibility responsibly; collaborate and work cooperatively with others; resolve conflicts; respond to moral and ethical challenges

Ethical comportment

Nursing education should prepare graduates to:

- Demonstrate self-awareness, self-care, self-growth; be open and non-judgmental
- Affirm and value diversity
- Appreciate the patient as a whole person, with his or her own life story and ideas about the meaning of health or illness
- Respect the patient's dignity, uniqueness, integrity, and self-determination, and his or her own power and self-healing processes
- Be open to others' ideas; show humility, mutual trust, empathy, support, and a capacity for grace

F. Teamwork

Teamwork is, appropriately, the final integrating concept in the NLN Education Competencies Model. Teamwork appears simple and self-evident; but it is crucial to each of the other five concepts and, ultimately, to patient outcomes. Consider the following:

- The IOM cites effective teamwork as the most important of its health care competencies in terms of ensuring quality and safety. Seventy percent of adverse events in health care settings, according to the IOM, are attributable to miscommunication and poor working relationships (IOM, 2003). *Relevant concept: Quality and safety.*
- The complex environment in which nurses work requires both intranursing and interprofessional teamwork to coordinate care across many disciplines (Apker, Propp, Zabava Ford, & Hofmeister, 2006). *Relevant concepts: Context and environment, Knowledge and science.*
- Including patients and families as team members can contribute to safer, more effective care (Sherwood, Thomas, Simmons, & Lewis, 2002). Relevant concepts: *Quality and safety; Relationship-centered care.*

- Poor teamwork is the leading factor in work dissatisfaction and contributes to high burnout and turnover (Sherwood, 2003). *Relevant concepts: Personal and professional development; Relationship-centered care.*

Effective communication is the foundation for effective teamwork (Haig, Sutton, & Whittington, 2006). Beyond communication skills, accomplished team members have a well-developed self-awareness (Horton-Deutsch & Sherwood, 2008) and can function alternately as leader, member, or follower, depending on the situation (e.g., the needs of the patient and family, competence of the primary health care provider, or the scope of practice). Contextual factors that contribute to poor teamwork include hierarchical reporting, authority gradients, frequent interruptions, multitasking, and work overload.

Mickan and Rodger (2005) developed a model characterizing effective health care teams. In their view, effective teams have:

- A well-defined *purpose*, relevant to patients and linked with their organization.
- *Goals* linked to the team's purpose and outcomes; these focus on the team's task.
- *Leadership* that influences activities toward goal achievement. Good leaders offer structured decision making. They help team members manage conflict and share ideas and information. They coordinate tasks, provide feedback, listen, and offer support and trust to team members.
- Regular patterns of *communication*. Effective communication is regular and consistent, so as to ensure the sharing of ideas and information, and at the same time flexible, so as to allow for diverse interpersonal skills.
- *Cohesion:* a sense of camaraderie and involvement generated from working together over time, participation in team tasks, and consistent communication. Cohesion builds commitment and trust, a shared pride in outcomes, and a desire to work together.
- *Mutual respect* between members. Team members are open to others' talents, beliefs, and professional contributions.

Students need opportunities in both simulation and guided clinical learning to practice team behaviors, to be prepared to navigate complex work settings, and to coordinate care using principles of delegation (Barnsteiner, Disch, Hall, Mayer, & Moore, 2007).

Teamwork means to function effectively within nursing and interprofessional teams, fostering open communication, mutual respect, and shared decision making to achieve quality patient care.

Apprenticeships for Teamwork

Knowledge

Nursing education should ensure graduates are familiar with concepts and literature in the following areas:

- Scope of practice, roles, and responsibilities of health care team members, including overlaps
- Contributions of other individuals and groups in helping patient/family achieve health goals
- Effective strategies for communicating with different members of the health team, including patients and families, nurses, and other health professionals
- Impact of team functioning on safety and quality of care, and how authority gradients influence teamwork and patient safety
- System barriers and facilitators of effective team functioning; strategies for improving systems to support team functioning

Practice

Nursing education should ensure graduates are able to:

- Act with integrity, consistency, and respect for differing views
- Function competently within one's own scope of practice as leader or member of the health care team and manage delegation effectively
- Clarify roles and integrate the contributions of others who play a role in helping the patient/family achieve health goals
- Adapt communication to the team and situation to share information or solicit input; initiate requests for help when appropriate
- Navigate conflict skillfully
- Choose communication styles that diminish the risks associated with authority gradients among team members to accomplish care, assert one's own views, and minimize risks associated with handoffs among providers and across transitions in care
- Participate in designing systems that support effective teamwork

Ethical comportment

Nursing education should prepare graduates to:

- Recognize the importance of one's own potential contribution to effective team functioning
- Value and respect the perspectives, attributes, and expertise of all health team members, including the patient/family
- Respect different styles of communication used by patients, families, and health care providers
- Recognize the risks across transitions in care and during handoffs among providers
- Value the influence of system solutions in achieving effective team functioning

Section V: Outcomes and Competencies

Program outcomes and core competencies in nursing education

As described in Section II of this document, the Work Group identified four broad outcomes applicable to all nursing programs. Graduates should be prepared (1) to promote and enhance *human flourishing* for patients, families, communities, and themselves; (2) to show sound *nursing judgment*; (3) to continually develop their *professional identity*; and (4) to maintain a *spirit of inquiry* as they move into the world of nursing practice, and beyond.

For clarity, we offer the following definitions. *Program outcomes* are defined as the expected culmination of all learning experiences occurring during the program, including the mastery of essential core nursing practice competencies, built upon the seven core values and six integrating concepts. *Course outcomes* are the expected culmination of all learning experiences for a particular course within the nursing program, including the mastery of essential core competencies relevant to that course. Courses should be designed to promote synergy and consistency across the curriculum and lead to the attainment of program outcomes.

Core competencies are the discrete and measurable skills, essential for the practice of nursing, that are developed by faculty in schools of nursing to meet established program outcomes. These competencies increase in complexity both in content and practice during the program of study. The core competencies are applicable in varying degrees across all didactic and clinical courses and within all programs of study, role performance, and practice settings. They structure and clarify course expectations, content, and strategies, and guide the development of course outcomes. They are the foundation for clinical performance examinations and the validation of practice competence essential for patient safety and quality care.

The tables presented on the following pages show, for each program outcome, the specific competencies expected of graduates of each program type. Importantly, the tables show how competencies build from one program type to the next, whereby the competencies for each program type reflect and assume mastery of those to their left in the tables. The tables thus graphically show the progression of knowledge, practice know-how, and ethical comportment across the programs, from a practical/vocational degree to a practice or research doctorate.

The various types of nursing education programs are defined in the second part of this section.

Program Outcome: Human Flourishing

Human flourishing is difficult to define, but it can be loosely expressed as an effort to achieve self-actualization and fulfillment within the context of a larger community of individuals, each with the right to pursue his or her own such efforts. The process of achieving human flourishing is a lifelong existential journey of hope, regret, loss, illness, suffering, and achievement. Human flourishing encompasses the uniqueness, dignity, diversity, freedom, happiness, and holistic well-being of the individual within the larger family, community, and population. The nurse helps the individual in efforts to reclaim or develop new pathways toward human flourishing.

Table 1

Graduate Competencies for Human Flourishing

PRACTICAL/ VOCATIONAL	ASSOCIATE DEGREE/ DIPLOMA	BACCALAUREATE	MASTER'S	PRACTICE DOCTORATE	RESEARCH DOCTORATE
Promote the human dignity, integrity, self-determination, and personal growth of patients, oneself, and members of the health care team.	Advocate for patients and families in ways that promote their self-determination, integrity, and ongoing growth as human beings.	Incorporate the knowledge and skills learned in didactic and clinical courses to help patients, families, and communities continually progress toward fulfillment of human capacities.	Function as a leader and change agent in one's specialty area of practice to create systems that promote human flourishing.	Systematically synthesize evidence from nursing and other disciplines and translate this knowledge to promote human flourishing within the organizational culture.	Design and implement research that promotes human flourishing of the nurse, nursing profession, patients, families, communities, populations, and systems.

Program Outcome: Nursing Judgment

Nursing judgment encompasses three processes: namely, critical thinking, clinical judgment, and integration of best evidence into practice. Nurses must employ these processes as they make decisions about clinical care, the development and application of research and the broader dissemination of insights and research findings to the community, and management and resource allocation.

Critical thinking means identifying, evaluating, and using evidence to guide decision making by means of logic and reasoning. Clinical judgment refers to a process of observing, interpreting, responding, and reflecting situated within and emerging from the nurse's knowledge and perspective (Tanner, 2006). Integration of best evidence ensures that clinical decisions are informed to the extent possible by current research (Craig & Smith, 2007).

Table 2

Graduate Competencies for Nursing Judgment

PRACTICAL/ VOCATIONAL	ASSOCIATE DEGREE/ DIPLOMA	BACCALAUREATE	MASTER'S	PRACTICE DOCTORATE	RESEARCH DOCTORATE
Provide a rationale for judgments used in the provision of safe, quality care and for decisions that promote the health of patients within a family context.	Make judgments in practice, substantiated with evidence, that integrate nursing science in the provision of safe, quality care and promote the health of patients within a family and community context.	Make judgments in practice, substantiated with evidence, that synthesize nursing science and knowledge from other disciplines in the provision of safe, quality care and promote the health of patients, families, and communities.	Make judgments in one's specialty area of practice that reflect a scholarly critique of current evidence from nursing and other disciplines and the capacity to identify gaps in knowledge and formulate research questions.	Systematically synthesize evidence from nursing and other disciplines and translate this knowledge to enhance nursing practice and the ability of nurses to make judgments in practice.	Provide leadership in designing and implementing research that expands the evidence underlying nursing practice and strengthens nurses' ability to make judgments.

Program Outcome: Professional Identity

Professional identity involves the internalization of core values and perspectives recognized as integral to the art and science of nursing. These core values become self-evident as the nurse learns, gains experience, and grows in the profession. The nurse embraces these fundamental values in every aspect of practice while working to improve patient outcomes and promote the ideals of the nursing profession. Professional identity is evident in the lived experience of the nurse, in his or her ways of "being," "knowing," and "doing."

Table 3

Graduate Competencies for Professional Identity

PRACTICAL/ VOCATIONAL	ASSOCIATE DEGREE/ DIPLOMA	BACCALAUREATE	MASTER'S	PRACTICE DOCTORATE	RESEARCH DOCTORATE
Assess how one's personal strengths and values affect one's identity as a nurse and one's contributions as a member of the health care team.	Implement one's role as a nurse in ways that reflect integrity, responsibility, ethical practices, and an evolving identity as a nurse committed to evidence-based practice, caring, advocacy, and safe, quality care for diverse patients within a family and community context.	Express one's identity as a nurse through actions that reflect integrity; a commitment to evidence-based practice, caring, advocacy, and safe, quality care for diverse patients, families, and communities; and a willingness to provide leadership in improving care.	Implement one's advanced practice role in ways that foster best practices, promote the personal and professional growth of oneself and others, demonstrate leadership, promote positive change in people and systems, and advance the profession.	As a nurse-scholar, seek ways to translate research findings into practice, and help design and implement changes in nursing practice and health policy that will best serve a diverse population and a diverse nursing workforce.	Implement one's role as a research scholar committed to a spirit of inquiry, the systematic investigation of nursing-related problems, and the dissemination of research findings, in a manner informed by a sense of responsibility to shape a preferred future for our profession.

Program Outcome: Spirit of Inquiry

A spirit of inquiry is a persistent sense of curiosity that informs both learning and practice. A nurse infused by a spirit of inquiry will raise questions, challenge traditional and existing practices, and seek creative approaches to problems. The spirit of inquiry suggests, to some degree, a childlike sense of wonder. A spirit of inquiry in nursing engenders innovative thinking and extends possibilities for discovering novel solutions in ambiguous, uncertain, and unpredictable situations.

Table 4

Graduate Competencies for Spirit of Inquiry

PRACTICAL/ VOCATIONAL	ASSOCIATE DEGREE/ DIPLOMA	BACCALAUREATE	MASTER'S	PRACTICE DOCTORATE	RESEARCH DOCTORATE
Question the basis for nursing actions, considering research, evidence, tradition, and patient preferences.	Examine the evidence that underlies clinical nursing practice to challenge the status quo, question underlying assumptions, and offer new insights to improve the quality of care for patients, families, and communities.	Act as an evolving scholar who contributes to the development of the science of nursing practice by identifying questions in need of study, critiquing published research, and using available evidence as a foundation to propose creative, innovative, or evidence-based solutions to clinical practice problems.	Contribute to the science of nursing in one's specialty area of practice by analyzing underlying disparities in knowledge or evidence; formulating research questions; and systematically evaluating the impact on quality when evidence-based solutions to nursing problems are implemented.	Disseminate practice-based knowledge by engaging in practice with an open mind; systematically studying the practice of other nurses; and reviewing extant research to formulate evidence-based proposals enhancing nursing practice, nursing education, or the delivery of nursing services.	Engage in the science of discovery by designing and implementing research studies and disseminating findings to improve nursing practice, nursing education, or the delivery of nursing services.

Educational Program Definitions, Outcomes, and Competencies

Here we present definitions of each program type, followed by statements of the competencies expected of graduates of such programs. The competencies for each program reflect and assume those addressed in any programs previously described.

Practical/Vocational Nursing Education

Practical or vocational nursing programs are approved schools that prepare and qualify graduates to take the NCLEX-PN (National Council Licensure Examination-Practical Nurse) exam. Upon receipt of their license, graduates are entitled to be called a Licensed Practical (or Vocational) Nurse (LPN/LVN) and to provide nursing care under the supervision of a Registered Nurse (RN). Many licensed practical and vocational nurses are employed in long-term care facilities, where they may be the main providers of day-to-day care. LPN/LVN programs are typically offered in technical schools, high schools, or community colleges, and they are usually 12 months in length, though they can vary from 10 to 18 months.

Competencies for Graduates of Practical/Vocational Programs

Human Flourishing
Promote the human dignity, integrity, self-determination, and personal growth of patients, oneself, and members of the health care team.

Nursing Judgment
Provide a rationale for judgments used in the provision of safe, quality care and for decisions that promote the health of patients within a family context.

Professional Identity
Assess how one's personal strengths and values affect one's identity as a nurse and one's contributions as a member of the health care team.

Spirit of Inquiry
Question the basis for nursing actions, considering research, evidence, tradition, and patient preferences.

Associate Degree Nursing Education

Associate degree (AD) nursing education provides the basic education necessary to become a registered nurse. Graduates are eligible to sit for the NCLEX-RN licensing examination and, if licensed, may practice in structured care settings, including hospitals, long-term care facilities, clinics, and offices. Associate degree nursing education incorporates nursing knowledge, knowledge of key biological and social sciences, and study of the humanities in a program that typically requires at least two years (65-75 credits) of study in a junior or community college.

Diploma Nursing Education

Diploma nursing programs have historically been based in hospitals, though today many affiliate with community colleges. These programs are two to three years in length, and upon completion, graduates earn a diploma in nursing, may earn an associate degree in science from an affiliating junior college, and are eligible to sit for the NCLEX-RN licensing examination. Like graduates of associate degree programs, graduates of diploma programs may work as RNs in structured care settings, including hospitals, long-term care facilities, clinics, and offices.

Competencies for Graduates of Associate Degree and Diploma Programs

Human Flourishing

Advocate for patients and families in ways that promote their self-determination, integrity, and ongoing growth as human beings.

Nursing Judgment

Make judgments in practice, substantiated with evidence, that integrate nursing science in the provision of safe, quality care and promote the health of patients within a family and community context.

Professional Identity

Implement one's role as a nurse in ways that reflect integrity, responsibility, ethical practices, and an evolving identity as a nurse committed to evidence-based practice, caring, advocacy, and safe, quality care for diverse patients within a family and community context.

Spirit of Inquiry

Examine the evidence that underlies clinical nursing practice to challenge the status quo, question underlying assumptions, and offer new insights to improve the quality of care for patients, families, and communities.

Baccalaureate Nursing Education

Baccalaureate nursing programs require a minimum of four years (120-135 credits) of study in a senior college or university, though some community colleges now offer baccalaureate programs. In addition to providing students with foundational knowledge and skills needed for practice as a registered nurse, baccalaureate nursing education includes learning experiences related to community and population-focused care, leadership and management, and research. Such programs also provide graduates with the foundation to enter graduate school, which, today, might be a master's program or a doctoral program.

Competencies for Graduates of Baccalaureate Programs

Human Flourishing
Incorporate the knowledge and skills learned in didactic and clinical courses to help patients, families, and communities continually progress toward fulfillment of human capacities.

Nursing Judgment
Make judgments in practice, substantiated with evidence, that synthesize nursing science and knowledge from other disciplines in the provision of safe, quality care and promote the health of patients, families, and communities.

Professional Identity
Express one's identity as a nurse through actions that reflect integrity, a commitment to evidence-based practice, caring, advocacy, and safe, quality care for diverse patients, families, and communities, and a willingness to provide leadership in improving care.

Spirit of Inquiry
Act as an evolving scholar who contributes to the development of the science of nursing practice by identifying questions in need of study, critiquing published research, and using available evidence as a foundation to propose creative, innovative, or evidence-based solutions to clinical practice problems.

Master's in Nursing Education

Master's-level nursing programs build and expand upon baccalaureate or entry-level nursing education, and they are designed to prepare individuals for advanced practice in a particular area of specialty. Such specialty roles include nurse practitioners, nurse anesthetists, clinical nurse specialists, nurse midwives, nurse educators, nurse administrators, clinical case managers, and nurse informaticists, among others. Master's-prepared nurses are expected to serve as leaders, members of interprofessional teams, and scholars who advance the profession, particularly in their chosen area of specialization.

NLN supports master's preparation for advanced practice nursing care in a reformed health care system and the role of master's education in preparing nursing administrators and nurse educators. At an Invitational Conference on Master's Education (given by the NLN in 2010), participants and panelists representing public and private nursing programs, nursing organizations, and advanced practice nursing programs, roles and practice environments confirmed the importance of embracing points of view that are inclusive of all nursing program types when addressing changes in advanced practice preparation. The model addresses this perspective and provides a strong foundation for present and future development of master's-prepared nurses.

Competencies for Graduates of Master's Programs

Human Flourishing
Function as a leader and change agent in one's specialty area of practice to create systems that promote human flourishing.

Nursing Judgment
Make judgments in one's specialty area of practice that reflect a scholarly critique of current evidence from nursing and other disciplines and the capacity to identify gaps in knowledge and formulate research questions.

Professional Identity
Implement one's advanced practice role in ways that foster best practices, promote the personal and professional growth of oneself and others, demonstrate leadership, promote positive change in people and systems, and advance the profession.

Spirit of Inquiry
Contribute to the science of nursing in one's specialty area of practice by analyzing underlying disparities in knowledge or evidence; formulating research questions; and systematically evaluating the impact on quality when evidence-based solutions to nursing problems are implemented.

Doctoral Nursing Education: Practice-Focused Doctorate

Doctoral programs in nursing and other practice disciplines can be categorized into two distinct types: practice-focused and research-focused.

Practice-focused doctoral programs are relatively new in nursing, and the essence of their focus continues to evolve. However, there is agreement that individuals who earn a practice doctorate are prepared to serve as leaders who promote and facilitate changes in practice that enhance the quality of care provided to individuals, families, and communities. Such change is grounded in sound evidence, enhanced by public policy initiatives, and reflective of a collaborative spirit among nurses and between nurses and other health professionals. Individuals who have earned a practice doctorate are considered to be the profession's most effective practice leaders, who will transform clinical practice.

Competencies for Graduates of a Practice Doctorate

Human Flourishing

Systematically synthesize evidence from nursing and other disciplines and translate this knowledge to promote human flourishing within the organizational culture.

Nursing Judgment

Systematically synthesize evidence from nursing and other disciplines and translate this knowledge to enhance nursing practice and the ability of nurses to make judgments in practice.

Professional Identity

As a nurse-scholar, seek ways to translate research findings into practice, and help design and implement changes in nursing practice and health policy that will best serve a diverse population and a diverse nursing workforce.

Spirit of Inquiry

Disseminate practice-based knowledge by engaging in practice with an open mind, systematically studying the practice of other nurses, and reviewing extant research to formulate evidence-based proposals enhancing nursing practice, nursing education, or the delivery of nursing services.

Doctoral Nursing Education: Research-Focused Doctorate

The majority of research-focused programs in nursing offer the academic doctorate, the PhD; however, some programs offer a professional doctorate, such as the DNS or DNSc. The research doctorate reflects preparation as a scientist, someone who designs and leads rigorous investigations into clinical practice, educational, system/administrative, or other issues in an effort to discover new knowledge and achieve new understandings. Such new knowledge provides the evidence that underlies nursing practice, identifies gaps in our knowledge, and serves to build the science of nursing.

Competencies for Graduates of a Research Doctorate

Human Flourishing

Design and implement research that promotes human flourishing of the nurse, nursing profession, patients, families, communities, populations, and systems.

Nursing Judgment

Provide leadership in designing and implementing research that expands the evidence underlying nursing practice and strengthens nurses' ability to make judgments.

Professional Identity

Implement one's role as a research scholar committed to a spirit of inquiry, the systematic investigation of nursing-related problems, and the dissemination of research findings, in a manner informed by a sense of responsibility to shape a preferred future for our profession.

Spirit of Inquiry

Engage in the science of discovery by designing and implementing research studies and disseminating findings to improve nursing practice, nursing education, or the delivery of nursing services.

Section VI: Competencies Survey

It was clear from the outset of this project that before any competencies or outcomes were finalized, the nursing education and practice communities would be asked to examine and comment on them. Toward this end, the Work Group prepared a survey designed to elicit feedback about the outcome and competency statements. Specifically, the survey was constructed to answer three main questions: (1) Are the four broad program outcome areas identified both valid and comprehensive? (2) Do the competency statements for each outcome successfully distinguish among the program types? (3) Do the competency statements accurately reflect what graduates of each program type ought to have achieved upon completion of the program?

As will be seen below, reaction to the outcome and competency statements was extremely positive. As a result, the statements presented in this monograph were altered only slightly from the forms they took in the survey.

Method

Instrument

The survey opened with a number of demographic questions (e.g., gender, ethnicity, education, and background in nursing practice). These were designed so the Work Group could check that the results reflected a reasonably representative sample of individuals from education and practice. The most relevant demographic data are given below, under Results.

The survey proper had five sections. In the first, respondents were given definitions of the four major outcome areas, and were asked to indicate the extent to which they thought each was a major outcome area for all nursing programs. Respondents answered this question on a Likert scale with five options, *Strongly agree, Agree, Disagree, Strongly disagree,* and *Don't know.* Respondents were also given the chance to make open-ended comments on any of the outcome areas or definitions at the end of the section.

The next two sections were designed in a similar manner. In the second section, respondents were given the competencies for each outcome along program type (that is, Tables 1 through 4 above). For each outcome, they were asked the extent to which they thought the competencies served to distinguish one program type from another.

In the third, the competencies were presented again, this time arranged according to program type; for each program type, respondents were asked the extent to which they thought graduates should be able to meet the competencies upon successful completion of such a program. In each case, the questions were answered along the same Likert scale used in Section 1, with a box for open-ended comments given at the section's end.

Sections four and five were designed to elicit respondents' overall perspective about the competencies and outcomes. In section four, respondents were asked to indicate their agreement (along the same Likert scale) with three statements: (1) The competencies reflect current practice for each program type; (2) The competency statements are clear; and (3) The outcomes require an appropriate degree of competency as students progress from one program type to the next. Again, a box at the end allowed for comments. Finally, section five included two open-ended questions: (1) What impact do the identified outcomes and competencies have for you and your program; and (2) How do these outcomes and competencies relate to practice, especially for new graduates?

Procedure

The Work Group prepared the survey for online distribution using Snap online survey software (www.snapsurveys.com). An invitation to participate in the survey was sent via email to all NLN members for whom valid email addresses were on file (about 31,000 individuals). It also was sent to non-NLN members in the NLN's database, and to 50 CEOs and presidents of practice organizations and other nursing organizations. Ultimately, the Work Group estimates that the invitation was issued to over 32,000 individuals, each of whom was encouraged to share the link with others. It is impossible to know exactly how many people saw the invitation or the survey. The survey was open for three weeks.

The Work Group received 1,309 completed surveys. The survey data were imported into SPSS data files at the Indiana University School of Nursing, where the consultant who was hired to complete the analysis was housed. The data were analyzed using descriptive statistics and thematic content analysis and were transformed in several ways prior to the final analyses. The open-ended comment sections of the survey resulted in more than 200 pages of data, which were analyzed collectively for their unique contribution.

Results

Demographics

Primary practice specialty. More than half the respondents belonged to one of three practice specialties: adult health/medical surgical (n = 336), acute/critical care (n = 253), and education (n = 127). The remaining respondents were divided among 23 other specialties.

Current nursing positions. The most frequently cited responses to this question were: nurse educator in an academic setting (n = 838), nurse educator in a practice setting (n = 434), administration (n = 285), consultant (n =127), staff nurse (n = 148), and clinical nurse specialist (n = 103). The total number of responses exceeds 1,309 (the number of respondents) because respondents were asked to check all positions that applied to them.

Program of primary teaching responsibility. This question was relevant only to the 838 respondents who identified themselves as nursing educators in an academic setting. Of the 837 who answered the question, the highest number were associate degree faculty (n = 380). Slightly over a quarter taught in baccalaureate programs (n = 230), and 84 in master's programs. Most of the remaining respondents were divided among practical/vocational (n = 45), diploma (n = 40), and doctoral (n = 25) programs. Four respondents checked "unknown/not applicable," and 29 checked "other."

Years as an RN. In the survey this variable was listed as "year of initial RN licensure"; it was changed for convenience prior to the analyses. Only 175 respondents answered this question. Among those who answered, years as an RN ranged from 1 to 56, with a mean of 29.69 years (SD = 9.85).

Highest nursing degree earned. The majority of respondents (n = 875) reported earning a master's as their highest nursing degree. Another 193 named the baccalaureate, and 189 had a doctorate. The remaining responses were divided among associate degree (n = 20), diploma (n = 8), practical/vocational diploma (n = 2), "unknown/not applicable" (n = 3), and "other" (n = 16). Three respondents did not answer this question.

Race/ethnicity/gender. The overwhelming majority of respondents (n = 1185) identified themselves as white. Fifty-nine identified themselves as black or African American, and small numbers as Asian (n = 23), American Indian or Alaska Native

(n = 16), Native Hawaiian or other Pacific Islander (n = 3), or "other" (n = 22). One respondent did not answer this question. Respondents were asked separately whether they identified themselves as Hispanic or Latino; at least 30 reported that they did so. Respondents were predominantly female (n = 1265); 40 were male; and four did not answer the gender question.

Competencies

In regard to the first section of the survey, nearly all respondents agreed or strongly agreed that the outcome areas presented are significant for all nursing programs. These figures, rounded to the nearest whole number, were 84 percent for human flourishing, 96 percent for nursing judgment, 94 percent for professional identity, and 92 percent for spirit of inquiry. The corresponding percentages of respondents who disagreed or strongly disagreed were 13 percent, 3 percent, 4 percent, and 7 percent, respectively. A small number of respondents marked the answer "Don't know" in response to this question. This figure was 1 percent or fewer for all the outcomes but human flourishing, where the "Don't know" option was chosen by 3 percent of respondents.

In the open comments part of section 1, some respondents expressed issues with aspects of a definition while not actually disagreeing that the outcome was important. Some comments suggest that respondents answered the question "should these be major outcomes" rather than the actual question of "to what extent are these major outcomes for nursing programs."

Generally, the comments were positive about all the outcomes. As the figures suggest, the only outcome that generated significant concern was human flourishing. Some respondents commented that human flourishing is a wonderful aspiration, something that is key to our professional development. Others felt the idea needed a different label or focus, needed to be broader in scope, or was perhaps too "existential."

With regard to section two, whether the competency statements for each outcome area "clearly distinguish one program type from another," there again was significant agreement, though not to the extent found for the previous section. For human flourishing, 77 percent of the respondents agreed or strongly agreed. These figures were 82 percent for nursing judgment, 80 percent for professional identity, and 83 percent for spirit of inquiry.

thoughtful comments. First, respondents were asked how they thought the outcomes and competency statements would affect them and their program. (The survey's instruction page directed respondents to understand "your program" as referring to the program in which they have the most extensive teaching, advisement, and leadership responsibilities.) Three major themes emerged in response to this question. (1) Many respondents indicated that their program would need to undergo curricular changes, including course outcomes, requiring preparation of faculty to address and measure these. (2) Many pointed out the difficulty of reconciling numerous and sometimes different standards (e.g., from the NLN, AACN, QSEN, CCNE [the Commission on Collegiate Nursing Education], and IOM). (3) Respondents suggested that clinical practices would need to revise their orientation programs, continuing education/staff development, and performance criteria. The comments suggested a general sense that the outcomes and competencies would raise the level of preparation and practice of all nurses, but that it would require a substantial time investment to achieve this goal.

The second of these questions asked respondents how the program outcomes and competency statements relate to practice, especially for new graduates. Two major themes emerged from the responses. Specifically, the outcomes and competencies were expected to bring about (1) increased accountability (particularly for evidence-based practice), and (2) clearer expectations and consistent standards regarding roles and the scope of practice for both nurses and employers.

Additional analyses

The Work Group conducted additional analyses to test for differences between respondents who were academicians and those who were not. In response to the survey's first question (are the outcome areas significant for all nursing programs), academicians had slightly higher agreement than non-academicians regarding human flourishing, nursing judgment, and professional identity, while non-academicians had slightly higher agreement vis-à-vis spirit of inquiry. Only with regard to professional identity was the difference statistically significant ($t = 3.52, p = .000$).

Analysis of all other quantitative questions revealed only one statistically significant difference, with regard to whether the competency statements reflect current practice for each program type (which, as noted above, received support from 80 percent of the respondents overall). Those working in academic settings showed greater agreement with this statement ($M = 2.26, SD = .96$) than non-academicians ($M = 2.4, SD = 1.03; t = 2.57, p = .01$). Other than this, no discernable patterns suggesting differences in perspective between the two sets of respondents were found.

Agreement with competency statements for each program type

As described above, the third section of the survey presented the competency statements for each program type, and respondents were asked the extent to which graduates of a given program should be able to meet the competencies for each outcome. This was an important question, as high levels of disagreement would have suggested that the competency statements did not reflect the real needs of the nursing community. In fact, the results were quite encouraging. As can be seen in the table below, all the competency statements but one received a minimum of 83 percent support ("agree" or "strongly agree"), and half received 90 percent or above. The only competency that received relatively low support (at 71 percent) was the spirit of inquiry competency for practical/vocational nurse education.

Table 5

Agreement with Competency Statements

Type of Program	Agreement with Competencies for Each Outcome[a]			
	Human Flourishing	Nursing Judgment	Professional Identity	Spirit of Inquiry
Practical/Vocational	85%	83%	85%	71%
Associate Degree/Diploma	90%	89%	89%	84%
Baccalaureate	91%	94%	93%	91%
Master's	93%	95%	95%	94%
Practice Doctorate	88%	89%	89%	89%
Research Doctorate	89%	91%	91%	90%

[a]Figures in the table represent percentage of all respondents who indicated they agree strongly agree that the competency statements reflect appropriate competencies for e program type and outcome.

Overall perceptions

In response to the three questions of section four, described above, 80 percen respondents agreed or strongly agreed that the competency statements reflect cur practice for each program type. Seventy-eight percent agreed or strongly agreed the competency statements were clear, and 73 percent that they build on each c from one program type to the next.

The two open-ended questions at the end of the survey, designed to elicit respond overall perceptions of the outcomes and competencies, brought forth a numb

Summary

It is evident from the survey findings that there is strong support for the four outcomes and accompanying competencies across all types of programs. This support indicates that these outcomes and competencies provide a valid and valuable framework for the ongoing development of nursing education programs. In addition, the similarity of responses from academicians and non-academicians suggests that collaboration of practice and academia in the preparation of nurses to meet the needs of patients, families, diverse populations, and communities in a reformed health care system is possible and desirable.

Those who practice in the academic world and those who practice in the care delivery world both view these outcomes and competencies as important guides for curriculum revision, staff development, faculty development, new nurse orientation, and progression along clinical ladders. It is hoped that both will continue to collaborate effectively in the education of nursing students, in developing multivariate approaches to measuring academic program outcomes, and in ensuring effective transitions from the student role to the role of clinician, advanced practice nurse, educator, administrator, informaticist, or scientist.

Section VII: Education and Practice Partnerships for the Future

The ideas presented in this document have evolved from rich discussions among nursing faculty, NLN leaders, nurse administrators, and nurses in staff development. All are agreed that we must redefine ourselves not through what divides us, but through what unites us. With this document, we affirm that education and practice are integral to each other, and it is in partnership that we can best serve our students, clients, practicing nurses, organizations, and communities.

The outcomes and integrating concepts of the NLN Education Competencies Model are applicable to all settings where nursing is practiced, from the clinical office (where the primary focus is the individual client's health) to administration (where the focus is the evolution or enhancement of health care systems). We hope that these outcomes and concepts will establish consistent baseline expectations about what students from all types of nursing programs are prepared to accomplish. We hope they will help graduates of all types of programs experience a smoother transition from the academic into the practice environment.

We further hope that the model will help experienced nurses within practice communities continue to participate in the moment of intersection between education and practice. Professional development specialists can build programs around these outcomes and integrating concepts to support the ongoing professional development of practicing nurses, so that the cycle of learning continues. We believe that the intersection between education and practice occurs at every moment that the nurse engages deeply in understanding his or her practice, and whenever conversations emerge among colleagues engaged in understanding how best to educate for and practice our discipline. Indeed, this goal is built into the model through its focus on evidence-based practice and the spirit of inquiry – concepts that we believe are among the most important innovations of the model.

Warner and Burton (2009) write about a new academic-service partnership constituted by a shared environment in which the worlds of academe and practice overlap; where joint scholarship and research, leadership development, and shared teaching support student development and create visions of lifelong learning for staff. In this environment, it is possible to imagine a shared world where practice partners help faculty shape and create curricula as well as clinical learning activities, and faculty participate in solving practice challenges and shaping and creating best practices in the service environment.

The following programs are offered as models for academic-practice partnerships in which academic faculty and practice partners come together to establish course goals, refine curricula, design clinical education models, and improve practice environments. The first example reports on a partnership among the University of Portland School of Nursing, in Portland, Oregon; Providence Health & Services (a not-for-profit health services network on the West Coast); and a US Veterans Administration facility to design and implement the Dedicated Education Unit (DEU) clinical education model. The second example describes a partnership between the Oregon Consortium for Nursing Education (OCNE) and practice partners throughout the state of Oregon to establish end-of-program competencies and develop, implement, and evaluate a new model of clinical education. The third example reports on the OCNE's partnership with various retirement homes and care centers in the Portland area to design and implement the Enriched Clinical Learning Environment through Partnerships in Long-Term Care (ECLEPs).

The DEU was inspired by a program developed in southern Australia and significantly adapted to fit within the American education and practice setting. The model involves an innovative partnership in which clinical units are devoted to the education of students and to the provision of excellent patient care within an active learning environment (Warner & Moscato, 2009). In this model, members of the clinical unit staff serve as clinical instructors for students, and university faculty serve as coaches to the nursing staff, helping develop their skills in clinical instruction. In addition to providing on-the-spot coaching, the university offers an orientation course for all new clinical instructors and continuing education for those already in the role. As the nurses and faculty adjust to the impact of staff nurses serving in clinical instructor roles, nurses develop a heightened sense of ownership and professionalism, while faculty are enriched by their new role as coaches. The model requires mutual respect, regular and open communication, and collaborative relationships, so that as challenges emerge, the faculty and clinical staff work together to develop improvements in the model (Moscato, Miller, Logsdon, Weinberg, & Chorpenning, 2007). The results are improved clinical education for students and the development of a dynamic learning community that engages and satisfies the nursing and interdisciplinary staff.

The Oregon Consortium for Nursing Education (OCNE) is a partnership among 13 Oregon Associate Degree and Baccalaureate Nursing Programs, led by the Oregon Health & Science University School of Nursing (OHSU). The programs share academic standards, common prerequisites, and co-admission for students to both community college and OHSU, so that students can complete coursework for a baccalaureate from OHSU without leaving their home community. The shared competency-based curriculum was designed through a multi-year collaborative process involving all OCNE partner campuses and representatives from hospitals, public health organizations, community agencies, and long-term care institutions (Gubrud & Schoessler, 2009; Tanner, Gubrud-Howe, & Shores, 2008). At the start of the process, participants were encouraged to form local faculty and practice teams to develop pilot projects that would test new and emerging clinical strategies. Six grant-supported pilot projects were selected from over 50 proposals submitted by the partner groups; these pilots helped inform the work of the clinical model design team. The final model was introduced in 2009 and is currently being studied in four OCNE campuses across the state. The model includes the development of Clinical Teaching Associate education programs for nursing staff who serve as clinical preceptors in the program.

The Enhancing Clinical Learning through Partnerships (ECLEPs) project evolved out of a need to prepare nurses with gerontologic expertise and to attract new nurses to community-based residential care and other long-term care (LTC) careers. ECLEPs addresses this need by fostering partnerships between academia and facilities that are "home" to older adults. ECLEPs create opportunities for faculty and staff nurses to develop relationships through workshops that address best practices in teaching and gerontologic nursing care. The workshops are highly interactive and designed so that faculty and staff nurses learn through and from each other. The workshops also give staff nurses the opportunity to interact with colleagues from other LTC settings, with the goal of developing a peer-support network. With feedback from staff nurses, faculty design student learning activities that address both course objectives and facility goals for excellence in care. The program's goals include encouraging students to see nursing in LTC settings as meaningful and challenging; to improve the care of older Oregonians; and to improve work environments in LTC so as to increase the recruitment and retention of nurses who desire to care for this population.

We hope that these examples will stimulate academic and practice partnerships which will create shared learning experiences that take nursing education and practice to a new place. Through a vibrant, dynamic interrelationship of practice and education we can together create our preferred future – preparing our students as practitioners in this exciting and challenging discipline, improving the practice environment to better support practitioners, and ensuring the best possible care for patients, families, and communities.

Section VIII: Implications of the Model for the Future of Nursing

Now is the time for transformation in nursing education. The word "transformation," by definition, suggests a significant change from a prior form or structure in response to a compelling stimulus. The dramatic complexity of the current health care environment – the explosion of scientific knowledge, the challenges of chronic disease management, the changing demography of the population, the changing roles of nurses, and escalating concerns surrounding the quality and outcomes of care – offer, we believe, more than sufficient stimulus to compel our community to radically reform nursing education.

Lewin (1951) conceptualized the experience of change as a process of *unfreezing*, followed by *movement and change* where new patterns and approaches are introduced, and culminating in a refreezing as the new patterns are accepted and become permanent. Transformation in nursing education is realized when faculty actively challenge the status quo and discard antiquated curricular practices (*unfreezing*), introduce innovative pedagogical frameworks and approaches (*movement and change*), and achieve widespread adoption and integration of new practices (*refreezing*). The model presented in this monograph provides a framework and support for authentic educational transformation in nursing.

This model is not intended to be prescriptive or dictatorial. Rather, it was intentionally constructed from a perspective of breadth and inclusivity that encourages schools of nursing to actively reflect on the expectations they articulate, the curricula and pedagogical practices designed to help students fulfill those expectations, and the educational experiences that will most effectively prepare students for contemporary practice. The model, therefore, supports the unique qualities and attributes that define each school. The possibilities afforded in the operationalization of this model are boundless.

The model employs a systems approach to education. The inputs, or the fundamental forces that permeate and inform the nursing educational program, are expressed in the core values that serve as guiding tenets for our profession. These core values must be integrated and developed in ways that are relevant to each specific nursing educational program. Questions related to the core values that faculty may want to consider as they apply the model include:

- What core values are appropriate for our nursing program? How do these tenets serve to distinguish the uniqueness of our program?
- How might we recognize, develop, and fully integrate the identified core values across our nursing education program?
- To what extent do our students reflect our core values? Should such values be addressed in the admission process and/or in the progression and graduation processes? What are the implications of this with respect to students?
- To what extent do our faculty reflect our core values? Should such values be addressed in the faculty search process and/or in our reappointment, promotion, and tenure processes? What are the implications of this with respect to faculty?
- To what extent are these core values congruent with the values expressed in our educational institution's mission statement?
- To what extent do our clinical partners reflect our identified values? To what extent have our collaborative efforts been congruent with the core values?
- What do we currently do that is not consistent with our core values? Is it time to discard and eliminate these inconsistent activities, practices, and orientations?

The *integrating concepts* reflect the throughputs in this systems model. Throughputs are woven throughout a system and provide essential integrity and cohesion. The six integrating concepts in the model are designed to be intentionally and progressively developed as students advance from one type of program to another and grow in their scope of responsibility. Questions related to the integrating concepts that faculty may want to consider as they apply the model include:

- What concepts are intentionally and progressively developed across the current curriculum at our school of nursing?
- How congruent are the concepts employed at our school of nursing with the six integrating concepts presented in the model?
- In what ways might our nursing program examine, reorganize, and appropriately incorporate the six integrating concepts?
- How are the apprenticeships of knowledge, practice, and ethical comportment realized for each concept identified in our nursing program?
- Are we teaching concepts or apprenticeships that are no longer relevant and therefore need to be eliminated from our curriculum?

Outcomes reflect the culmination of complex, multifaceted learning, which can be demonstrated at the time of program completion. Educational outcomes are mediated by their unique integration and interpretation on the part of each individual nurse graduate. Questions related to outcomes that faculty may want to consider as they apply the model include:

- What outcomes are formally identified for our school of nursing?
- How congruent are the articulated outcomes for our school of nursing with the four outcomes espoused in this model?
- Does our school of nursing currently uphold outcomes that are no longer relevant and therefore need to be eliminated from the program?
- In what ways might our nursing program examine, reorganize, and appropriately incorporate the four outcomes in this model?

The *competencies* are discrete and identifiable skills essential for the practice of nursing. Competency statements reflect the degree preparation and role performance expected of the graduate. Questions related to the competencies that faculty may want to consider as they apply the model include:

- What competencies are formally identified for graduates of our school of nursing?
- How congruent are the identified competencies for our school of nursing with the competencies articulated in this model?
- Does our school of nursing currently uphold competencies that are no longer relevant and therefore need to be eliminated?

Nursing education has "tinkered around the edges" of real curricular reform for decades. Indeed, were faculty to merely layer the ideas presented in the model on top of an existing program of study, they would only serve to actualize the well-documented phenomenon of the "additive curriculum" (Diekelmann, 1992), and fail to transform nursing education in any substantive way. The time is now for faculty in schools of nursing to gather, reflect, zestfully investigate, debate, and engage in comprehensive redesign of the curriculum in nursing. This model provides a framework to enact this long-envisioned educational transformation. Our students, the public we serve, and the profession of nursing deserve nothing less.

Section IX: Recommendations for Future Work

The following recommendations are offered for nurse educators, nursing faculty administrators, nurses in practice settings, regulators, nursing accreditation bodies, and the NLN itself. Through these recommendations, we hope the Education Competencies Model presented in this monograph can become a true force for change.

For Nurse Faculty

- Develop assessment methods to measure student attainment of the competencies reflected in the NLN Education Competencies Model.
- Develop program outcomes and level/course/unit objectives that reflect the uniqueness of a particular school and that are congruent with the outcomes identified in the model.
- Design innovative curricula, teaching strategies and evaluation methods that align with stated program outcomes, level/course/unit objectives, and the model.
- Propose ways in which faculty can contribute to the development of the science of nursing education and promote evidence-based teaching practices that will most effectively help students achieve the outcomes identified in the model.
- Create partnerships with practice colleagues to design new curriculum models and classroom/clinical learning experiences that will enable students to achieve the program outcomes identified in the model.
- Encourage students to continue academic progression and lifelong learning that enables them to expand their competencies and implement new roles as noted in the model.
- Seek input from students to determine the relevance of the model to them and the kind of learning experiences they believe would best enable them to meet the program outcomes identified in it.

For Deans/Directors/Chairpersons

- Initiate discussions among faculty, with clinical partners and other stakeholders, and across the nursing education community regarding curriculum reform inspired by the NLN Education Competencies Model and the program outcomes and competencies it includes.

- Partner with practice colleagues to design creative collaborative initiatives to assure graduates are prepared to practice in current and future practice environments.
- Partner with other nursing programs to create innovative and expanded pathways for academic progression.
- Involve colleagues from practice settings in the school's advisory, curriculum, or other committee/board where they can have input regarding future directions of the school and how students are educated.
- Foster a healthful work environment and support faculty though curriculum reform inspired by the model and the program outcomes and competencies it includes.
- Champion multisite pedagogical research initiatives designed to test and evaluate the model.

For Practice Settings

- Partner with academic colleagues to develop transition-to-practice models that build on the outcomes articulated for various types of programs.
- Develop programs and initiatives that support the ongoing academic progression of staff, enabling them to expand their competencies and implement new roles as noted in the NLN Education Competencies Model.
- Create partnerships with academic colleagues in the design of new curriculum models, classroom/clinical learning experiences, and evaluation methods that will enable students to achieve the program outcomes identified in the model.
- Provide access to clinical settings appropriate for testing aspects of the model.

For Regulators (legal and voluntary)

- Explore ways to best align licensure processes and requirements with the program outcomes articulated in the NLN Education Competencies Model.
- Ensure that the licensing examination is aligned with the program outcomes articulated in the model.
- Encourage innovation in curriculum models, classroom/clinical learning experiences, and evaluation methods that are designed collaboratively by academic/practice partnerships to reflect concepts included in the model.

For Nursing Accreditation Bodies

- Develop accreditation standards for each type of nursing program that reflect the program outcomes, competencies, and integrating concepts identified in the NLN Education Competencies Model.

- Articulate the uniqueness of preparation in various types of nursing programs.

For the National League for Nursing

- Provide faculty development opportunities designed to help faculty in all types of programs create new curriculum models, classroom/clinical learning experiences, and evaluation methods that are congruent with the program outcomes, competencies, and integrating concepts inherent in the NLN Education Competencies Model.
- Partner with colleagues in education and practice settings to develop and implement research protocols to test the model.
- Provide funds and secure external funding to support testing and ongoing refinement of the model.
- Incorporate the model in the NLN's publications, faculty excellence initiatives, and future strategic efforts.
- Use a variety of means to disseminate results of pilot projects, evaluation studies, and other projects that will help nursing faculty and clinical partners apply and further develop the model.

Appendix A

Members of the NLN Educational Competency Work Group

June Larson, MS, RN, CNE, ANEF, (NEAC Member 2006, NEAC Chair, 2007-2009)

Marilyn Brady, PhD, RN (NEAC Member, 2008-2010)

Carol Coose, EdD, RN, CNE (NEAC Chair-elect, 2007-2009 & Chair, 2009-2011)

Lynn Engelmann, EdD, RN, CNE, ANEF (NEAC Member, 2008-2011)

Linda Everett, PhD, RN, NEA-BC, FAAN (Practice Colleague, 2008-2010)

Karen Pardue, MS, RN, CNE, ANEF (NEAC Member, 2007-2010)

Mary Schoessler, EdD, RN-BC (Practice Colleague, 2008-2010)

Gwen Sherwood, PhD, RN, FAAN (Practice Colleague, 2008-2009)

Theresa ("Terry") Valiga, EdD, RN, ANEF, FAAN (Nurse Educator Colleague, 2008-2010)

Kynna Wright, PhD, MPH, RN, CPNP (NEAC Chair-elect, 2009-2011)

Brother Ignatius Perkins, OP, PhD, RN, FAAN, FNYAM (NLN Board of Governors Liaison to NEAC, 2007-2011)

Cathleen Shultz, PhD, RN, CNE, FAAN (NLN President-elect, 2007-2009: President, 2009-2011)

Janice Brewington, PhD, RN, FAAN (NLN Chief Program Officer & Liaison to Work Group, 2009; NLN Senior Director for Professional Development, 2010)

Mary Anne Rizzolo, EdD, RN, FAAN (NLN Senior Director for Professional Development & Liaison to Work Group, 2008-2009)

Stacey Schrand, BFA (NLN Committee Coordinator & Support for Work Group, 2008-2010)

Note: The NEAC is the Nursing Education Advisory Council, an executive committee of the NLN. This elected group of individuals is charged with responsibility to provide the leadership that transforms nursing education and supports innovation in all types of nursing education programs to achieve excellence and prepare graduates for practice in the 21st century.

Appendix B
Subconcepts for Context and Environment

Ambiguity and Uncertainty

Ambiguity and uncertainty are part of the human condition. Despite the explosion of knowledge that helps define the modern age, much of the world remains unknown. Perhaps nowhere is this more evident than in health care, where the individuals, families, groups, and communities for whom professionals care are complex, unpredictable systems; where the health conditions being addressed are complex phenomena; and where responses to interventions are influenced by the uniqueness of each human being. Nurses and other health care providers must become comfortable with this lack of certainty, and must learn to accept, manage, and even benefit from it. Indeed, ambiguity and uncertainty can be frightening, but they may also encourage creativity, innovation, and risk taking.

Global Health

The concept of global health underscores the interconnectedness of all people and places. Global health approaches emphasize culturally competent care delivered within accessible, integrated care systems. Global health incorporates aspects of population-based health promotion, environmental health, transmission of disease, management of chronic illness, health policy, and health care economics. Global health is not defined in a geographic sense, but is rather a lens that extends across localities, regions, nations, and the world.

Health Care Economics

Economics is the study of how scarce resources are allocated among their possible users. As a management or policy tool, economics is used to ensure that individuals, organizations, and societies make optimal use of limited resources. Health care economics is the study of the actions and behaviors of patients, third-party payers – including the government – and providers of health care services in the allocation of scarce resources (Finkler, Kovner, & Jones, 2007). Within nursing, health care economics means examining the cost/benefit ratio of health care by endeavoring to answer five questions: 1) What will be produced? (What is the desired goal of health care?) 2) How will the output be produced? (What is needed to reach the desired health care outcome?) 3) How much will be produced? (How much health care will be available?) 4) Who will get the output produced? (Who will have access to available health care?) and 5) Who will produce the output? (Who will provide the needed health care services?) The answers must be informed by an understanding of factors related to resource utilization (safety, effectiveness, cost, and impact on practice in the planning and delivery of health care services) as well as the impact of public policy on access to health care and the structure of health care delivery systems.

Healthful Work Environments

Healthful workplace/educational environments for nurses and nursing students incorporate several essential competencies. They require effective and open communication; active relationship-centered collaboration; competent and credible nurse/faculty leadership; recognition and respect for the value of nurse/student contributions; accountability; and the encouragement of continued professional growth and development.

Informatics

Informatics is a broad term encompassing information science and information technologies. Briefly put, it involves the design, development, use, and management of computer-based information systems. In nursing, informatics is becoming increasingly important in every sphere, from patient care to systemwide operations to research. In general, nurse informaticist competencies can be divided into three major areas: 1) direct care (care management, clinical decision making, operations management, communication); 2) support (clinical support, measurement, analysis, research and reports, administrative and financial); and 3) information infrastructure (security, health record management, registry and directory services, terminology services, standards-based interoperability, business rules management, and workflow management) (TIGER Informatics Competencies Team, 2008).

Innovation and Creativity

The NLN Work Group on Innovation in Nursing Education (NLN, 2005) defined innovation as using knowledge to create ways and services that are new (or perceived as new) to transform systems. Innovation requires deconstructing or challenging long-held assumptions and values. The outcome of innovation in nursing education is excellence in nursing practice and development of a culture that supports risk taking, creativity, and excellence (Pardue, Tagliareni, Valiga, Davison-Price, & Orehowsky, 2005).

Leadership

In nursing, leadership can be defined as the ability and willingness to articulate a vision of a preferred future for the profession or some area of nursing practice; to enlist others to "join in the journey" to realize that vision; to take risks to create new practices or policies in that area; and to facilitate change, manage conflict, and help others grow in their own leadership potential.

Systems Thinking

Systems thinking in nursing emphasizes the examination of patterns and relationships within the unpredictable and chaotic environment of health care delivery. The process of systems thinking affirms the interconnectedness of people, roles, relationships and functions, and the interdependence of each on the other. Systems thinking seeks to facilitate interdisciplinary team functioning, reduce risks, identify areas for improvements, and support optimal health outcomes.

Appendix C

The NLN Science of Nursing Education Model

The NLN's Science of Nursing Education Model (NLN, 2003), adapted and shown below, illustrates the many activities that must be undertaken to develop a science and the many ways in which members of a discipline can fulfill their responsibility to contribute to the ongoing evolution of that body of knowledge.

The stimulus for creating the Science of Nursing Education Model came from evidence-based reform needs in practice and education. The model is a first-ever conceptual illustration of the numerous processes involved in building a science. That process is a nonlinear, iterative process in which all activities noted in the model need to occur and each can be conducted simultaneously (Shultz, 2009).

If graduates of basic and advanced nursing programs are to provide the leadership needed to deliver quality care, promote the health of our nation, and create a preferred future for the profession, then practice initiatives and educational programs need to be innovative, flexible, and responsive to change. To make wholesale change based on "hunches," "popular trends," or "gut feelings" is not defensible. Instead, change must arise from what has been learned through research.

Such research in nursing education is called pedagogical research, and is conducted by scholars in numerous fields of nursing. The research identifies the most effective approaches to help students achieve desired learning outcomes for providing quality care to individuals, families, and communities, and for advancement of the profession. With increasing expectations that graduates use evidence-based practice, the teaching and learning of that practice also must be evidence-based. It is no longer enough to hope that nursing students learn what they need to know to practice nursing. Instead nurse educators must use teaching and evaluation strategies that research demonstrates have the most success achieving desired learning outcomes (Gresley, 2009).

The science of nursing education can be guided by the nursing education research priorities formulated by the NLN (2008), available at http://www.nln.org/research/priorities.htm. Practice research priorities are identified through various organizations, including the National Institute of Nursing Research. Research priorities help a profession's members clarify the gaps in knowledge that need scholarly attention so those gaps can be addressed and the practice of that profession can be evidence-based.

Figure 2

Science of Nursing Education Model

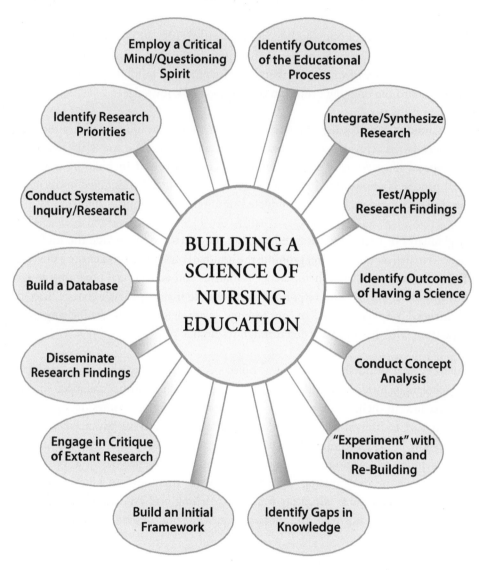

Shultz, C. (Ed.) (2009). Building a science of nursing education: Foundation for evidence-based teaching-learning. New York: National League for Nursing.

Appendix D
Glossary

Caring means "promoting health, healing, and hope in response to the human condition."

"A culture of caring, as a fundamental part of the nursing profession, characterizes our concern and consideration for the whole person, our commitment to the common good, and our outreach to those who are vulnerable. All organizational activities are managed in a participative and person-centered way, demonstrating an ability to understand the needs of others and a commitment to act always in the best interests of all stakeholders" (NLN, 2007).

Context and Environment, in relation to organizations, refer to the conditions or social system within which the organization's members act to achieve specific goals. Context and environment are a product of the organization's human resources, and also the policies, procedures, rewards, leadership, supervision, and other attributes that influence interpersonal interactions. In health care, context and environment encompass organizational structure, leadership styles, patient characteristics, safety climate, ethical climate, teamwork, continuous quality improvement, and effectiveness.

Core Competencies are the discrete and measurable skills, essential for the practice of nursing, that are developed by faculty in schools of nursing to meet established program outcomes. These competencies increase in complexity both in content and practice during the program of study. The core competencies are applicable in varying degrees across all didactic and clinical courses and within all programs of study, role performance, and practice settings. They structure and clarify course expectations, content, and strategies, and guide the development of course outcomes. They are the foundation for clinical performance examinations and the validation of practice competence essential for patient safety and quality care.

Course Outcomes are the expected culmination of all learning experiences for a particular course within the nursing program, including the mastery of essential core competencies relevant to that course. Courses should be designed to promote synergy and consistency across the curriculum and lead to the attainment of program outcomes.

Diversity means recognizing differences among "persons, ideas, values and ethnicities," while affirming the uniqueness of each.

"A culture of diversity embraces acceptance and respect. We understand that each individual is unique and recognize individual differences, which can be along the dimensions of race, ethnicity, gender, sexual orientation, socioeconomic status, age, physical abilities, religious beliefs, political beliefs, or other ideologies. A culture of diversity is about understanding ourselves and each other and moving beyond simple tolerance to embracing and celebrating the richness of each individual. While diversity can be about individual differences, it also encompasses institutional and systemwide behavior patterns" (NLN, 2007).

Excellence means "creating and implementing transformative strategies with daring ingenuity."

"A culture of excellence reflects a commitment to continuous growth, improvement, and understanding. It is a culture where transformation is embraced, and the status quo and mediocrity are not tolerated" (NLN, 2007).

Ethics involves reflective consideration of personal, societal, and professional values, principles and codes that shape nursing practice. Ethical decision making requires applying an inclusive, holistic, systematic process for identifying and synthesizing moral issues in health care and nursing practice, and for acting as moral agents in caring for patients, families, communities, societies, populations, and organizations. Ethics in nursing integrates knowledge with human caring and compassion, while respecting the dignity, self-determination, and worth of all persons.

Holism is the culture of human caring in nursing and health care that affirms the human person as the synergy of unique and complex attributes, values, and behaviors, influenced by that individual's environment, social norms, cultural values, physical characteristics, experiences, religious beliefs and practices, and moral and ethical constructs within the context of a wellness-illness continuum.

Human Flourishing can be loosely expressed as an effort to achieve self-actualization and fulfillment within the context of a larger community of individuals, each with the right to pursue his or her own such efforts. The process of achieving human flourishing is a lifelong existential journey of hope, regret, loss, illness, suffering, and achievement. Human flourishing encompasses the uniqueness, dignity, diversity, freedom, happiness, and holistic well-being of the individual within the larger family, community, and population. The nurse helps the individual in efforts to reclaim or develop new pathways toward human flourishing.

Integrity means "respecting the dignity and moral wholeness of every person without conditions or limitation."

"A culture of integrity is evident when organizational principles of open communication, ethical decision making, and humility are encouraged, expected, and demonstrated consistently. Not only is doing the right thing simply how we do business, but our actions reveal our commitment to truth telling and to how we always were ourselves from the perspective of others in a larger community" (NLN, 2007).

Knowledge and Science refer to the foundations that serve as a basis for nursing practice, which, in turn, deepen, extend, and help generate new knowledge and new theories that continue to build the science and further the practice. Those foundations include (a) understanding and integrating knowledge from a variety of disciplines outside nursing that provide insight into the physical, psychological, social, spiritual, and cultural functioning of human beings; (b) understanding and integrating knowledge from nursing science to design and implement plans of patient-centered care for individuals, families, and communities; (c) understanding how knowledge and science develop; (d) understanding how all members of a discipline have responsibility for contributing to the development of that discipline's evolving science; and (e) understanding the nature of evidence-based practice.

Nursing Judgment encompasses three processes: namely, critical thinking, clinical judgment, and integration of best evidence into practice. Nurses must employ these processes as they make decisions about clinical care, the development and application of research and the broader dissemination of insights and research findings to the community, and management and resource allocation.

Critical thinking means identifying, evaluating, and using evidence to guide decision making by means of logic and reasoning. Clinical judgment refers to a process of observing, interpreting, responding, and reflecting situated within and emerging from the nurse's knowledge and perspective (Tanner, 2006). Integration of best evidence ensures that clinical decisions are informed to the extent possible by current research (Craig & Smith, 2007).

Patient-Centeredness is an orientation to care that incorporates and reflects the uniqueness of an individual patient's background, personal preferences, culture, values, traditions, and family. A patient-centered approach supports optimal health outcomes by involving patients and those close to them in decisions about their clinical care. Patient-centeredness supports the respectful, efficient, safe, and well-coordinated transition of the patient through all levels of care.

Personal and Professional Development is a lifelong process of learning, refining, and integrating values and behaviors that (a) are consistent with the profession's history, goals, and codes of ethics; (b) serve to distinguish the practice of nurses from that of other health care providers; and (c) give nurses the courage needed to continually improve the care of patients, families and communities and to ensure the profession's ongoing viability.

Professional Identity involves the internalization of core values and perspectives recognized as integral to the art and science of nursing. These core values become self-evident as the nurse learns, gains experience, and grows in the profession. The nurse embraces these fundamental values in every aspect of practice while working to improve patient outcomes and promote the ideals of the nursing profession. Professional identity is evident in the lived experience of the nurse, in his or her ways of "being," "knowing," and "doing."

Program Outcomes are the expected culmination of all learning experiences occurring during the program, including the mastery of essential core nursing practice competencies, built upon the seven core values and six integrating concepts.

Quality and Safety is the degree to which health care services 1) are provided in a way consistent with current professional knowledge; 2) minimize the risk of harm to individuals, populations and providers; 3) increase the likelihood of desired health outcomes; and 4) are operationalized from an individual, unit, and systems perspective.

Relationship-Centered Care positions (a) caring; (b) therapeutic relationships with patients, families, and communities; and (c) professional relationships with members of the health care team as the core of nursing practice. It integrates and reflects respect for the dignity and uniqueness of others, valuing diversity, integrity, humility, mutual trust, self-determination, empathy, civility, the capacity for grace, and empowerment.

Spirit of Inquiry is a persistent sense of curiosity that informs both learning and practice. A nurse infused by a spirit of inquiry will raise questions, challenge traditional and existing practices, and seek creative approaches to problems. The spirit of inquiry suggests, to some degree, a childlike sense of wonder. A spirit of inquiry in nursing engenders innovative thinking and extends possibilities for discovering novel solutions in ambiguous, uncertain, and unpredictable situations.

Teamwork means to function effectively within nursing and interprofessional teams, fostering open communication, mutual respect, and shared decision making to achieve quality patient care.

Bibliography

All Nursing Schools: Your Guide to Nursing Education and Careers [Directory website]. (2002-2010). Retrieved from http://www.allnursingschools.com/faqs/programs

American Association of Colleges of Nursing. (2004). Position statement on the practice doctorate in nursing. Retrieved from http://www.aacn.nche.edu/DNP/DNPPositionStatement.htm

American Association of Colleges of Nursing. (2008). The essentials of baccalaureate education for professional nursing practice. Retrieved from http://www.aacn.nche.edu/Education/pdf/BaccEssentials08.pdf

American Association of Colleges of Nursing. (2010). The essentials of master's education in nursing [Draft]. Retrieved from http://www.aacn.nche.edu/Education/pdf/DraftMastEssentials.pdf

American Nurses Association. (2010). Promoting healthy work environments: A shared responsibility. Retrieved from http://www.nursingworld.org/MainMenuCategories/ANAMarketplace/ANAPeriodicals/OJIN/JournalTopics/Promoting-Healthy-Work-Environments.aspx

American Nurses Association. (2004). *Nursing: Scope and standards of practice* (4th ed.). Silver Spring, MD: Author.

Armstrong, G. E., Spencer, T. B., & Lenburg, C. B. (2009). Using quality and safety education for nurses to enhance competency outcome performance assessment: A synergistic approach that promotes patient safety and quality outcomes. *Journal of Nursing Education, 48*(12), 686-693.

Bargagliotti, L. A., & Lancaster, J. (2007). Quality and safety education in nursing: More than new wine in old skins. *Nursing Outlook, 55*, 156-158.

Barrett, E. A. (2002). What is nursing science? *Nursing Science Quarterly, 15*(1), 51-60.

Begley, A. M. (2006). Facilitating the development of moral insight in practice: Teaching ethics and teaching virtue. *Nursing Philosophy, 7*, 257-265.

Brown, S. J. (2008). *Evidence-based nursing: The research-practice connection.* Sudbury, MA: Jones & Bartlett.

Burkemper, J., Dubois, J., Lavin, M. A., Meyer, G. A., & McSweeney, M. (2007). Ethics in education in MSN programs: A study of national trends. *Nursing Education Perspectives, 28*(1), 10-17.

Carper, B. (1978). Fundamental patterns of knowing in nursing. *Advances in Nursing Science, 1*(1), 13-23.

Carter, K. F., Kaiser, K. L., O'Hare, P. A., & Callister, L. C. (2006). Use of PHN competencies and ACHNE essentials to develop teaching-learning strategies for generalist C/PHN curricula. *Public Health Nursing, 23*(2), 146-160.

Cassidy, L., & Bardon, C. (2006). One year after the AACN standards: Where are we now? *AACN Advanced Critical Care, 17*(2), 119-124.

Clegg, S., & Hardy, C. (Eds.). (1999). *Studying organizations: Theory and method.* Thousand Oaks, CA: Sage.

Consensus Panel on Genetic/Genomic Nursing Competencies. (2009). *Essentials of genetic and genomic nursing: Competencies, curricula guidelines, and outcome indicators* (2nd ed.). Silver Spring, MD: American Nurses Association.

Dickenson-Hazard, N. (2004). Global health issues and challenges. *Journal of Nursing Scholarship, 36*(1), 6-10.

Dixon, J., Larison, K., & Zabari, M. (2006). Skilled communication: Making it real. *AACN Advanced Critical Care, 17*(4), 376-382.

Doane, G., Pauly, B., Brown, H., & McPherson, G. (2004). Exploring the heart of ethical nursing practice: Implications for ethics education. *Nursing Ethics, 11*(3), 240-253.

Dossey, B. (2007). Theory of integral nursing guidelines. Retrieved from http://www.dosseydossey.com/barbara/pdf/Dossey_Theory_of_Integral_Nursing_PPT_Guidelines.pdf

Driever, M. J. (2002). Are evidence-based practice and best practice the same? *Western Journal of Nursing Research, 24*(5), 591-597.

Duffy, J., & Hoskins, L. (2003). The Quality-Caring Model©: Blending dual paradigms. *Advances in Nursing Science, 26*(1), 77-88.

Falk-Rafael, A. (2006). Globalization and global health: Toward nursing praxis in the global community. *Journal of Advanced Nursing, 29*(1), 2-14.

Fawcett, J. (2000). The state of nursing science. Where is the nursing in the science? *Theoria: Journal of Nursing Theory, 9*(3), 3-10.

Fawcett, J. (2005). *Contemporary nursing knowledge: Analysis and evaluation of nursing models and theories* (Rev. ed.). Philadelphia: F. A. Davis.

Fitzpatrick, J. (2003). Nurses as healers [Editorial]. *Nursing Education Perspectives, 24*(3), 117.

Fontaine, D., & Gerardi, D. (2005). Healthier hospitals. *Nursing Management, 36*(10), 34-44.

Gardner, J. W. (1989). The tasks of leadership. In W. E. Rosenbach & R. L. Taylor (Eds.), *Contemporary issues in leadership* (2nd ed., pp. 24-33). Boulder, CO: Westview Press.

Garman, A. N., Burkhart, T., & Strong, J. (2006). Business knowledge and skills: Competencies. *Journal of Healthcare Management, 51*(2), 81-85.

Gerardi, D., & Fontaine, D. (2007). True collaboration: Envisioning new ways of working together. *AACN Advanced Critical Care, 18*(1), 10-14.

Grossman, S. G., & Valiga, T. M. (2009). *The new leadership challenge: Creating the future of nursing* (3rd ed.). Philadelphia: F. A. Davis.

Halstead, J. A. (Ed.). (2007). *Nurse educator competencies: Creating an evidence-based practice for nurse educators.* New York: National League for Nursing.

Hegyvary, S. T. (2004). Working paper on grand challenges in improving global health. *Journal of Nursing Scholarship, 36*(2), 96-100.

Hodson Carlton, K., Ryan, M., Ali, N. S., & Kelsey, B. (2007). Integration of global health concepts in nursing curricula: A national study. *Nursing Education Perspectives, 28*(3), 124-129.

Holden, L. M. (2005). Complex adaptive thinking: A concept analysis. *Journal of Advanced Nursing, 52*(6), 651-657.

Hughes, R. (Ed.) (2008). *Patient safety and quality: An evidence-based handbook for nurses.* (Agency for Healthcare Research and Quality (AHRQ) Publication No. 08-0043). Retrieved from http://www.ahrq.gov/qual/nurseshdbk/

Huston, C. (2008). Preparing nursing leaders for 2020. *Journal of Nurse Management, 16*, 905-911.

Ireland, M. (2008). Assisting students to use evidence as a part of reflection on practice. *Nursing Education Perspectives, 29*(2), 90-93.

Jackson, A., Dowell, M., Steele, E., & Faller, H. (1997). Health partnerships: Learning and sharing. *Journal of Nursing Education, 36*(6), 252-255.

Kelley, R. (1992). *The power of followership: How to create leaders people want to follow and followers who lead themselves.* New York: Currency Doubleday.

Kerfoot, K., & Lavandero, R. (2005). Healthy work environments: Enroute to excellence. *Critical Care Nurse, 25*(3), 71-72.

Kramer, M., & Schmalenberg, C. (2008a). Confirmation of a healthy work environment. *Critical Care Nurse, 28*(2), 56-64.

Kramer, M., & Schmalenberg, C. (2008b). The practice of clinical autonomy in hospitals: Twenty thousand nurses tell their story. *Critical Care Nurse, 28*(6), 58-71.

Lenburg, C. B., Klein, C., Abdur-Rahman, V., Spencer, T. B., & Boyer, S. (2009). The COPA model: A comprehensive framework designed to promote quality care and competence for patient safety. *Nursing Education Perspectives, 30*(5), 312-317.

Leners, D., Roehrs, C. & Picone, A. (2004). Tracking the development of professional values in undergraduate nursing students. *Journal of Nursing Education, 46*(12), 504-511.

Lindley, D. (2008). *Uncertainty: Einstein, Heisenberg, Bohr, and the struggle for the soul of science.* New York: Knopf Publishing Group.

Malloch, K. (2001). Assessing your organization's leadership development: Systems thinking. *Patient Care Management, 16*(10), 8-11.

Manojlovich, M., & DeCicco, B. (2007). Healthy work environments, nurse-physician communication, and patients' outcomes. *American Journal of Critical Care, 16*(6), 536-543.

Mark, B., Hughes, L., Belyea, M., Bacon, C., Chang, Y., & Jones, C. (2008). Exploring organizational context and structure as predictors of medication errors and patient falls. *Journal of Patient Safety, 4*(2), 66-77.

Marx, D. (2001). Patient safety and the "just culture": A primer for health care executives. Retrieved from http://psnet.ahrq.gov/resource.aspx?resourceID=1582

Massey, Z., Rising, S. S., & Ickovics, J. (2006). Centering pregnancy group prenatal care: Promoting relationship-centered care. *Journal of Obstetric, Gynecologic and Neonatal Nursing, 35*(2), 286-294.

McCauley, K. (2005). A message from the American Association of Critical-Care Nurses. *American Journal of Critical Care, 14*(3), 186.

McLeroy, K. (2006). Thinking of systems. *American Journal of Public Health, 96*(3), 402.

Melnyk, B. M., & Fineout-Overholt, E. (2005). *Evidence-based practice in nursing and healthcare: A guide to best practice.* Philadelphia: Lippincott, Williams & Wilkins.

Messias, D. K. H. (2001). Globalization, nursing and health for all. *Journal of Nursing Scholarship, 33*(1), 9-11.

Murray, J. P. (2004). The globalization of nursing for a healthy world. *Nursing Education Perspectives, 25*(4), 158.

National Association for Associate Degree Nursing. (2010). Position statements. Retrieved from https://www.noadn.org/component/option,com_docman/Itemid, 250/task,cat_view/gid,87/

National League for Nursing. (2005). Core competencies of nurse educators. Retrieved from http://www.nln.org/facultydevelopment/pdf/corecompetencies.pdf

National League for Nursing. (2009). The NLN Healthful Work Environment Tool Kit ©. Retrieved from http://www.nln.org/facultydevelopment/HealthfulWork Environment/index.htm

Nightingale Initiative for Global Health. (n.d.). Retrieved July 9, 2008, from http:// www.nightingaledeclaration.net/ndc/

Nolan, M., Keady, J., & Aveyard, B. (2001). Relationship-centered care is the next logical step. *British Journal of Nursing, 10*(12), 757.

Northouse, L., & Northouse, P. (1998). *Health communications: Strategies for health professionals.* Stamford, CT: Appleton & Lange.

Outcome Engineering. (2008). The Just Culture Algorithm, (Version 3.0) [Computer software]. Plano, TX: Author.

Pearson, A., Wiechula, R., & Lockwood, C. (2007). A re-consideration of what constitutes 'evidence' in the healthcare professions. *Nursing Science Quarterly, 20*(1), 85-88.

Penz, K. L., & Bassendowski, S. L. (2006). Evidence-based nursing in clinical practice: Implications for nurse educators. *Journal of Continuing Education in Nursing, 37*(6), 250-254.

Pittman, T. S., Rosenbach, W. E., & Potter, E. H., III. (1998). Followers as partners: Taking the initiative for action. In W. E. Rosenbach & R. L. Taylor (Eds.), *Contemporary issues in leadership* (4th ed., pp. 107-120). Boulder, CO: Westview Press.

Pravikoff, D. S., Tanner, A. B., & Pierce, S. T. (2005). Readiness of U.S. nurses for evidence-based practice. *American Journal of Nursing, 105*(9), 40-51.

Puchalski, C., & McSkimming, S. (2006). Creating healing environments. *Health Progress, 87*(3), 30-35.

Rycroft-Malone, J., Seers, K., Tichen, A., Harvey, G., Kitson, A., & McCormack, B. (2004). What counts as evidence in evidence-based practice? *Journal of Advanced Nursing, 47*(1), 81-90.

Sadler, J. (2003). A pilot study to measure the caring efficacy of baccalaureate nursing students. *Nursing Education Perspectives, 24*(6), 295-299.

Safran, D., Miller, W., & Beckman, H. (2006). Organizational dimensions of relationship-centered care: Theory, evidence and practice. *Journal of General Internal Medicine, 21*(S1), S9-S15.

Schmidt, N. A., & Brown, J. M. (2009). *Evidence-based practice for nurses: Appraisal and application of research.* Sudbury, MA: Jones & Bartlett.

Shirey, M. (2006). Authentic leaders creating healthy work environments for nursing practice. *American Journal of Critical Care, 15*(3), 256-268.

Simmons, J. (Ed.). (1993). *Prospectives: Celebrating 40 years of associate degree nursing education.* New York: National League for Nursing Press.

Skiba, D. J. (2005). Preparing for evidence-based practice: Revisiting information literacy. *Nursing Education Perspectives, 26*(5), 310-311.

Steefel, L. (2005). AACN issues call to action for healthy work environment. *Nursing Spectrum – Midwest Edition, 6*(3), 21.

Stetler, C. (2003). The role of the organization in translating research into evidence-based practice. *Outcomes Management for Nursing Practice, 7*(3), 97-103.

Stevens, K. R. (2002). *ACE Star Model of EBP: The cycle of knowledge transformation.* San Antonio, TX: Academic Center for Evidence-Based Practice

Thornby, D. (2006). Beginning the journey to skilled communication. *AACN Advanced Critical Care, 17*(3), 266-271.

Torrance, E. P. (1979). *The search for Satori and creativity.* Buffalo, NY: Creative Education Foundation.

Triola, N. (2006). Dialogue and discourse: Are we having the right conversations? *Critical Care Nurse, 26*(1), 60-66.

Triola, N. (2007). Authentic leadership begins with emotional intelligence. *AACN Advanced Critical Care, 18*(3), 244-247.

Verhey, M. P. (1999). Information literacy in an undergraduate nursing curriculum: Development, implementation and evaluation. *Journal of Nursing Education, 38*(6), 252-259.

Watson, J. (2005). [Commentary on Nurse-patient interaction: A review of the literature, by M. Shattell, *Journal of Clinical Nursing 13*, 714-722.]. Journal of Clinical Nursing, 14(4), 530-533.

White, J. L. (2005). Introducing undergraduate students to global health challenges through web-based learning. *Nursing Education Perspectives, 26*(3), 157-162.

Zipperer, L., & Tompson, S. (2006). Systems thinking. *Information Outlook, 10*(12), 16-20.

References

American Association of Colleges of Nursing. (1996). *The essentials of master's education for advanced practice nursing.* Washington, DC: Author.

American Association of Colleges of Nursing. (1998). *The essentials of baccalaureate education for professional nursing practice.* Washington, DC: Author.

American Association of Critical-Care Nurses. (2005). AACN standards for establishing and sustaining healthy work environments: A journey to excellence. *American Journal of Critical Care, 14*(3), 187-197. [Standards available at www.aacn.org/hwe].

American Nurses Association. (2003). *Nursing's social policy statement* (2nd ed.). Washington, DC: Author.

American Nurses Association. (2005). *Code of ethics for nurses with interpretive statements.* Retrieved from http://nursingworld.org/ethics/code/protected_nwcoe813.htm

American Nurses Association. (2006). *Essential nursing competencies and curricula guidelines for genetics and genomics.* Silver Spring, MD: Author.

Apker, J., Propp, K., Zabava Ford, W., & Hofmeister, N. (2006). Collaboration, credibility, compassion, and coordination: Professional nurse communication skill sets in health care team interactions. *Journal of Professional Nursing, 22*(3), 180-189.

Barnsteiner, J., Disch, J., Hall, L., Mayer, D., & Moore, S. (2007). Promoting interprofessional education. *Nursing Outlook, 55*(3), 144-150.

Benner, P., Sutphen, M., Leonard, V., & Day, L. (2009). *Educating nurses: A call for radical transformation.* San Francisco: Jossey-Bass.

Blau, P., & Scott, W. (1962). *Formal organizations.* San Francisco: Chandler.

Craig, J. V., & Smith, R. (2007). *The evidence-based practice manual for nurses* (2nd ed.). Philadelphia: Churchill Livingstone Elsevier.

Cronenwett, L., Sherwood, G., Barnsteiner, J., Disch, J., Johnson, J., Mitchell, P., et al. (2007). Quality and safety education for nurses. *Nursing Outlook, 55*(3), 122-131.

Diekelmann, N. (1992). Learning-as-testing: A Heideggerian hermeneutical analysis of the lived experiences of students and teachers in nursing. *Advances in Nursing Science, 14,* 72-83.

Donaldson, L. (1999). The normal science of structural contingency theory. In S. Clegg & C. Hardy (Eds.), *Studying organizations: Theory and method* (pp. 51-70). Thousand Oaks, CA: Sage.

Etzioni, A. (1964). *Modern organizations.* Englewood Cliffs, NJ: Prentice-Hall.

Finkler, S. A., Kovner, C. T., & Jones, C. B. (2007). *Financial management for nurse managers and executives.* St. Louis, MO: Saunders Elsevier.

Gresley, R. S. (2009). Building a science of nursing education. In C. M. Shultz (Ed.), *Building a science of nursing education* (pp. 1-13). New York: National League for Nursing.

Gubrud, P., & Schoessler, M. (2009). OCNE Clinical Education Model. In N. Ard & T. Valiga (Eds.), *Clinical nursing education: Current reflections* (pp. 39-58). New York: National League for Nursing.

Haig, K., Sutton, S., Whittington, J. (2006). SBAR: A shared mental model for improving communication between clinicians. *Journal of Quality Patient Safety, 32*(3), 167-175.

Halstead, J. A. (Ed.). (2007). *Nurse educator competencies: Creating an evidence-based practice for nurse educators.* New York: National League for Nursing.

Horton-Deutsch, S., & Sherwood, G. (2008). Reflection: An educational strategy to develop emotionally competent nurse leaders. *Journal of Nursing Management, 16,* 946-954.

Ingersoll, G. L. (2000). Evidence-based nursing: What it is and what it isn't. *Nursing Outlook, 48,* 151-152.

Institute of Medicine. (2001). *Crossing the quality chasm: A new health care system for the 21st century.* Washington, DC: National Academy of Sciences. [Executive summary available at http://www.iom.edu/Reports/2001/Crossing-the-Quality-Chasm-A-New-Health-System-for-the-21st-Century.aspx]

Institute of Medicine. (2003). *Health professions education: A bridge to quality.* Washington, DC: National Academies Press.

International Council of Nurses. (2006). *ICN code of ethics for nurses.* Retrieved November 1, 2008, from http://www.icn.ch/icncode.pdf

Lewin, K. (1951). *Field theory in social science.* New York: Harper and Row.

Massachusetts Organization of Nurse Executives. (2007). *Nurse of the future: Nursing core competencies* [Draft #2]. Retrieved from http://www.mass.edu/currentinit/documents/NursingCoreCompetencies.pdf

Mickan, S., & Rodger, S. (2005). Effective health care teams: A model of 6 characteristics developed from shared perceptions. *Journal of Interprofessional Care, 19*(4), 358-370.

Mitchell, P. (2008). Defining patient safety and quality care. In R. Hughes (Ed.), *Patient safety and quality: An evidence-based handbook for nurses.* (Agency for Healthcare Research and Quality (AHRQ) Publication No. 08-0043). Retrieved from http://www.ahrq.gov/qual/nurseshdbk/docs/MitchellP_DPSQ.pdf

Moscato, S., Miller, J., Logsdon, K., Weinberg, S., & Chorpenning, L. (2007). Dedicated education unit: An innovative clinical partner education model. *Nursing Outlook: 55*(1), 31-37.

National League for Nursing. (2003). *Building the science of nursing education model.* New York: Author.

National League for Nursing. (2005). Core competencies of nurse educators. Retrieved from http://www.nln.org/facultydevelopment/pdf/corecompetencies.pdf

National League for Nursing. (2007). NLN core values. Retrieved from http://www.nln.org/aboutnln/corevalues.htm

National League for Nursing. (2008). Research priorities in nursing education. Retrieved from http://www.nln.org/research/priorities.htm.

Oregon Consortium for Nursing Education. (2007). Competency rubrics and benchmarks [Provisional]. Retrieved from http://www.ocne.org/competencies.html

Pardue, K. T., Tagliareni, M., Valiga, T., Davison-Price, M., & Orehowsky, S. (2005). Substantive innovation in nursing education: Shifting the emphasis from content coverage to student learning. [Headlines from the NLN]. *Nursing Education Perspectives, 26*(1), 55-57.

Rathert, C., & Fleming, D. (2008). Hospital ethical climate and teamwork in acute care: The moderating roles of leaders. *Health Care Management Review, 33*(4), 323-331.

Sherwood, G. (2003). Leadership for a healthy work environment: Caring for the human spirit. *Nurse Leader, 1*(5), 36-40.

Sherwood, G., & Drenkard, K. (2007). Quality and safety curricula in nursing education: Matching practice realities. *Nursing Outlook, 55*, 151-155.

Sherwood, G., Thomas, E., Simmons, D., & Lewis, P. (2002). A teamwork model to promote patient safety in critical care. *Critical Care Nursing Clinics of North America, 14*, 333-340.

Shultz, C. (Ed.). (2009). *Building a science of nursing education: Foundation for evidence-based teaching-learning.* New York: National League for Nursing.

Tanner, C. A. (2006). Thinking like a nurse: A research-based model of clinical judgment in nursing. *Journal of Nursing Education, 46*(6), 204-211.

Tanner, C. A., Gubrud-Howe, P., & Shores, L. (2008). The Oregon Consortium for Nursing Education: A response to the nursing shortage. *Policy, Politics and Nursing Practice, 9*(3). 203-209.

TIGER Informatics Competencies Team. (2008). Tiger competencies: Basic computer, information literacy, and information management/informatics competencies. Retrieved April 24, 2008, from http://tigercompetencies.pbwiki.com

Tresolini, C. P., & the Pew-Fetzer Task Force. (1994). *Health professions education and relationship-centered care.* San Francisco, CA: Pew Health Professions Commission.

Warner, J., & Burton, D. (2009). The policy and politics of emerging academic-service partnerships. *Journal of Professional Nursing, 25*(6), 329-334.

Warner, J., & Moscato, S. (2009). An innovative approach to clinical education: Dedicated education units. In N. Ard & T. Valiga (Eds.), *Clinical nursing education: Current reflections* (pp. 59-70). New York: National League for Nursing.